A Safe Place
For Mama

by

Gladys Kepney White

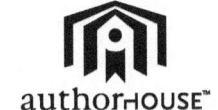

authorHOUSE™

1663 LIBERTY DRIVE, SUITE 200
BLOOMINGTON, INDIANA 47403
(800) 839-8640
WWW.AUTHORHOUSE.COM

AuthorHouse™
1663 Liberty Drive, Suite 200
Bloomington, IN 47403
www.authorhouse.com
Phone: 1-800-839-8640

AuthorHouse™ UK Ltd.
500 Avebury Boulevard
Central Milton Keynes, MK9 2BE
www.authorhouse.co.uk
Phone: 08001974150

First published by AuthorHouse 6/9/2006

ISBN: 1-4208-9616-4 (sc)

Library of Congress Control Number: 2005909975

*Printed in the United States of America
Bloomington, Indiana*

This book is printed on acid-free paper.

Cover Design By: Joannah Seaborn

*Scripture quotations are taken from the Hebrew/Greek
Keyword Study Bible, unless otherwise indicated.*

Dedicated to My Mother:
Teacher Leona Kepney

In Memory of My Father:
Deacon William Kepney

October 2002

TABLE OF CONTENTS

Acknowledgements.. ix

Foreword... xi

Author's Preface... xiii

Introduction: The Disease.................................... xxiii

01. She Lost Her Mind?... 1

02. Mama 13

03. Bill.. 25

04. The Children 37

05. The Church 47

06. Beliefs 57

07. Standards.. 65

08. Communication 79

09. Healing & Peace 101

10. The Mind: A Terrible Thing to Lose 115

11. My Mother/My Friend.................................... 119

12. What Do We Do With Mama? 125

13. The Conclusion of the Matter....................... 135

Appendix: Tips for Communication 145

ACKNOWLEDGEMENTS

To **James**, my faithful husband,
Eboni, **J. Harris** (Nicole) and **Jeryme**,
(The best children in all the earth).
I love you more than you will ever know!

To **Wilma**, **Darrell** and **Trish,** my siblings, without
whom this book would not be possible.
I love you guys dearly.

To **Bishop Joseph & Teacher Linda Phillips**,
thanks for accepting me into the Nazaree Family. I
have grown by leaps and bounds.
Thank you so much.

To **Elder Margaret Curry** who has provided me with an accelerated study of God's word. You are my Biblical mentor. Thank you.

To **Mrs. Brenda E. Rocker** who encouraged me to complete this product. You are a Godsend.

To **Joel**, **Eboni Nikol**, **Patricia** & **Vicki** who corrected my 'wrongs'. You are a very important part of this assignment.
Bless You!

And

To **All** those who trust God and have loved ones that have fallen victim to this disease.

FOREWORD

Into every life there comes crisis that we are not prepared to handle; neither can education prepare us for these experiences.

It is daily living through problems, step by step, that patience becomes experience and experience brings knowledge, which helps the family understand and accept the suffering of their loved one after the onset of such conditions.

Alzheimer's is such a sickness. It brings into a family many situations beyond their control. Yet, it gives them an appreciation for the good days of the past.

This book gives us a glimpse into the heart of a loving daughter. Her feelings are easily perceived by the reader.

Gladys shares her childhood memories with love and humor. She attributes the Scriptures as the source of her strength. She is a woman of integrity whom I have known professionally and spiritually for many years. Her assignment from God with **FAVOR** Ministries, Inc has truly equipped her to have empathy with those who suffer in diverse situations.

Reverend Margaret L. Curry
President & Founder of Citadel of Hope Bible Institute

AUTHOR'S PREFACE

Alzheimer's disease is a devastating illness of the mind. It removes its victim from life as they know it; from understanding to confusion, from clarity to bewilderment. Strangely enough, it brings both tears and laughter to the caretakers. Tears are shed because there is a sense of loss and confusion as the person affected is still alive with reasonable health right in your presence, but seemingly so far away. Laughter is brought on by some of the conversations that are entered into by that person who is just trying to get a simple thought across. This book is written to bring comfort to those who have experienced the effects of a loved one who has fallen prey to this dreadful disease. It is to encourage the faithful and bring some understanding of just who God is to the unbeliever in this type of situation.

If you believe in the Bible and trust that what it says is both true and for our good, this book is for you. If you need a little humor while you are going through with a loved one, this book is for you. If you find yourself at a loss as to whether the next step is acceptance or denial, this book is for you. If you do not believe in the Bible and need someone to explain the works of God and what is said in His Word regarding healing, this book is definitely for you.

My siblings, my father and I were at a standstill as to how to receive what was happening to our mother and his wife. It affected not only our mother, but also each of us in many ways. At the onset, it was devastating. Why her? We all found ourselves in a state of denial. We did not want this to happen to her. The person that we leaned on could no longer hold a straight conversation with us. We could no longer call and get advice. Instead, we had to make the decisions for her. Funny, when we were growing up she would go down the list of each of our names to get to the one she actually wanted. She would say, "Wilma, Darrell, Patricia Lynette, I mean Gladys. You know who you are, come here." This was when things were good and she knew who we were. It would upset us because she could not immediately recall our names, but she would eventually get to it. Now, as the Alzheimer's has progressed, she really has forgotten who we are. She may go through that same list and never get to our name. Now she calls us names that belong to her siblings.

How can we get through to her? Where has she gone? Beyond that beautiful silver gray hair is a well of knowledge. There lay a plethora of revelation of the Word of God. Experiences were accumulated for more than 75 years. Information contained was "how to": how to raise children, how to keep a husband, how to cook hot water corn bread. We should have been busy writing and learning what she knew. How I wish we had known how important that information would be to us. So much was hidden, could it all be lost? We asked the question, how could we tap into that mind? We wanted her back with all the memories, the experiences, the information and the revelations.

My brother, Darrell, said the most difficult hour for him was at the initial doctor's visit. During testing, Mama answered so many questions correctly. She spelled familiar words like 'world' and spelled it backwards. Because she answered so many correctly, Darrell felt a little hope; a possible light at the end of the tunnel. Maybe, this was just a temporary thing. She may have gotten her medicine confused and took too much and it caused this interruption of her thought pattern. Surely there is an explanation for such a brilliant mind to suddenly go blank. Then there was the bombshell. She was told to repeat the words 'cat, rat and hat' and she could not do it. This confirmed an overwhelming truth.

Shortly after that a lighter side manifested. While visiting Mama in the nursing home, my brother was able to see humor in this debilitating disease. When talking with her, she kept calling him Leroy although his name is Darrell. Leroy is actually her brother;

our uncle. He told her, "Mama, I'm Darrell, not Uncle Leroy." She continued to call him Leroy. He kept saying "My name is Darrell." After several rounds of this, she finally asked him, "Well, when did you change your name?" He had to laugh.

Destiny

There is comfort in knowing that we serve a God who is Omniscient, Omnipresent, and Omnipotent. He is a God who knows all, is everywhere and has all power. He knows our journey. He knows His thoughts toward us, and they are thoughts of peace and not evil to get us to an expected end. He knows what vehicle we will take to remove us from this earth, and He knows when we should board that vehicle. He determines whether the ride should be a short trip or a lengthy journey. He knows how to protect us from the evil that is to come. He knows just how much we can bear. God has the power to accomplish it all. It is our duty to trust Him. What a Mighty God we serve!

To know God is to accept His will for our lives even when we have messed up the plan. He knows how to orchestrate the symphony of our lives even when the tuba player quits, the cellist is not present or the percussionist is on his way. Our job is to sit in our respective places and wait on the instructions. The music sheet (God's Word) is placed on the stand right before our eyes. We just have to make sure that we are familiar with the music. We trust that the Conductor knows when to bring us in and when to keep us silent. Sometimes we just have to mark time. The crescendos, decrescendos and the pauses are a part of the symphony. Harmony must be established or the music does not flow. Music from all of the instruments can be blended so that it will appear to be only one sound, but everyone must be directed or there will be utter chaos. The conductor is an extremely important part of the concert. He brings order. The sheet music may be in place, the musicians in their chairs, the microphones adjusted and the crowd waiting, but if the Conductor is not present all is in vain.

God is the Conductor of the Christian life. He keeps the symphony in tune and the music flowing. When one part of our lives gets off track or out of tune, God knows just how to bring us back into harmony. He keeps our instruments in order. *Colossians 1: 17* – "And he is before all things, and by him all things consist." The word "consist" in the Greek is the word 'sunistemi' which means "in Him are all things held together." Christ keeps us together. In the midst of our trials he keeps us together. When the peace in our lives is missing, Jehovah Shalom -the God of Peace- steps in to keep us together. The adversary throws his best punches and yet we bounce back, because the Creator, the Almighty God has promised to keep us 'held together'.

Externally, Mama's situation seems confused, but if we are to believe the Word of God we can rest assured that He is still in control. He is holding her peace and her spirit together. Our prayer is that He keeps her in perfect peace. We have known some patients to be combative, but Mama keeps the jovial spirit that she exhibited before this change. This is God letting us know that through these circumstances He is yet God and in control. In Him all things <u>do</u> consist. The Jesus that she knew before any physical changes occurred is still the same. He is immutable; He changes not. Hold fast to what you believe in God. Let no circumstances or temporary situations change your faith in God. We firmly believe that God keeps her at peace and He 'holds her together'.

Mama has always been a fighter. She is by nature a tough character; a strong spirit. She would pretty much let you know what was on her mind and there was no doubt as to what she meant. The concerts of life had made her defensive. She would have to play unfamiliar instruments. In spite of it all she kept the music playing.

Now, things have slightly changed. A new score of music is before us, but the Conductor is still the same. A fiery spirit is now docile. It is hard to believe, but the tough character has mellowed into a calm sweet spirit. God has brought her to a place of peace where she does not to have to fight for her chair anymore. She does not have to be on the defense. We accept this quiet spirit as her original personality. She is now a person we miss, but at the same time we are glad she has returned to who she really is.

If you are experiencing a loved one, friend or family member going through this stage of their lives, I pray that this book brings comfort to you. Enjoy the humor, accept the reality and feel the love. Just knowing that there are others who have similar situations should bring some ease to your mind that you are not alone. This book should bring some clarity as you strive to make good decisions. Your first and last consultant should be God – in all thy ways acknowledge him and he will direct your path *(Proverbs 3:6)*.

INTRODUCTION
The Disease

Alzheimer's is a dreadful disease. It robs us of people we know without physically taking them from us. It is said that the mind is a terrible thing to waste, but it is also a terrible thing to lose. It is terrible not just for the person attacked, but for the people who love and care for the well being of the victim. Only our faith in God can sustain us through that which we don't understand. Our trust in the Almighty helps us to keep a grip on the handlebars of life. When it appears that it is better to let go, God wants us to "hold on because help is on the way."

FACTS:

Alzheimer's is a common form of dementia. Dementia is a group of disorders in which progressive destruction of brain cells leads to an increasingly severe decline in memory, thinking and reasoning.

About 4 million people in the United States have Alzheimer's. It is an illness that makes it difficult for its victim to recall recent events, rationalize and use their vocabulary. It can cause strange reactions to situations and moodiness in the individual. Eventually, people with Alzheimer's have a hard time with every day chores such as using the telephone, cooking or handling money.

The disease primarily strikes older adults. It affects all races. Ten percent of individuals over 65 and nearly 50 percent of people over 85 are likely to be affected. It is believed to arrive from a combination of genetic and non-genetic factors rather than from any single cause. Although there is no single test to detect the disorder, physicians are now able to diagnose Alzheimer's disease with an accuracy rate above 90 percent. We do not know how to prevent it or cure it, but successful treatment is more effective when begun in the early stages.

DETECTION:

There is no single test to detect Alzheimer's. General testing may take more than one day. It may include a visit to a primary care physician along with consultations with specialist such as psychiatrist or neurologist. A medical history is taken, complete physical, neurological examination, laboratory tests, a brain imaging procedure and evaluation of mental status as well as a psychiatric assessment. [1]

PROGNOSIS:

Isaiah 53:5 – "But He was wounded for our transgressions, He was bruised for our iniquities: the chastisement of our peace was upon him, and with His stripes we are healed."

---

[1] 2003 Alzheimer Disease and Related Disorders Association, Inc.

CHAPTER I
She Lost Her Mind?

Towards the end of the year 2001, a drastic change occurred that caught the Kepney family off guard. We were not prepared for the change and therefore had difficulty adjusting to it. We had lost jewelry, money, directions, friends and even loved ones, but never in our wildest dreams did we fathom one of us losing our ability to reason. The warning was so subtle that we nearly missed it, but as we reflect on past events, the signs were clear, but so easily ignored. Because we are God-fearing people, we were able to cope and look to God for answers. Mama was changing. Change interrupts patterns, rituals, habits and norms. Pieces of the puzzle no longer fit properly, perhaps because the edges are torn. To live with the change we, my father, siblings and myself, had to accept the inevitable. We had to accept the fact, without an explanation of why, that one of us was changing. Those pieces were not going to fit anymore no matter how hard we shoved. What do we do? How do we pray? What do we pray for? Mama was changing.

Isaiah 57:1 – "The righteous perisheth, and no man layeth it to heart: and merciful men are taken away, none considering that the righteous is taken away from the evil to come." When we enter a secret place with God and remain, we never know the pain that He may be sparing us. We often ask for healing for our sick loved ones, not realizing that healing is also in death. To be absent from the body is to be present with the Lord. In his presence there is fullness of joy – no pain, no hurting, no depression, but fullness of joy. Because Mama's mind is in that, secret place, she has not witnessed the sorrows of this present age. She did not understand what happened on September 11, 2001. She does not know about the war in Iraq. The tsunami means nothing to her. Gas prices are not her concern. She will never know that gas is over $2.60 a gallon. Katrina is just another child's name. Her secret place keeps her in peace. That is what we pray for her: 'peace' and that is what she receives from God. Medical science prefers we believe that Mama's brain is shrinking and daily losing function. They say that memory lost will never be recovered. They may be right to a point, but they do not have the last say. I choose to believe that even though the conversation has changed, because she cannot convey thoughts as clearly as before, the memories of a good life are stored somewhere inside her. God, who is just so good, will allow her to photo play a picture at any time. Every now and then, she brings up an event that we have forgotten, but she still recalls. The long time memory lets me know that it is still there. We hear it when she mentions her own mother, who has been deceased since 1987. We see it as out of place when she mentions her name, but she sees it as it was. She actually remembers our names, but finds it difficult to call them when we are present. Who is to say that our names are not in a **'Safe Place**'?

Knowing that the *'Safe Place'* may exist comforts us when we look at a face whose expression has not changed, but whose words are jumbled. She has a face that still warms us with a comforting look. We can see beyond the bewilderment and remember what once was. We can still see wisdom, intelligence, temperance and love. It is as if she is always saying, "Baby, it's all right. Mama still loves you." At an initial visit when she was first placed in a nursing home, I could not help but cry because of the turn of events. She calmly looked at me and asked, "Why are you crying?" "Everything is fine." I had no answer. Then I thought if you are at peace, I should be also.

She lost her mind?

Where is her mind? Is it locked in some secret place in her heart? Is it stored in a safe place in the back of her head? Where is it? How can we find it? Is it in some place hidden from even her, but a safe place? Could it be in a place where memories do not fade, but are tucked away for rainy days? Like a safe with a combination that only the owner knows the right numbers to turn and set to open at will. Is there a secret passage to the past where memories are never lost, just stored for keep sakes?

We are partially responsible for what is placed in our 'Safe Place'. What we do and say all adds up and is placed in the folder. If we choose to do good things, they are placed in the folder. If we choose to do bad things then they are likewise stored. It behooves us to check just what we are putting in our 'Safe Place'. How we live now may be very important as to how we live later.

Memories are brought up at strategic times:

❖ Memories of cool days of summer and cuddling days of winter; Of leaves falling in autumn and flowers blooming in spring

❖ Memories of hot homemade biscuits covered with real Karo syrup straight from the can

❖ Memories of safe days when only a little metal latch was necessary to safe guard a home

❖ Memories of bare feet on hot concrete not bothered by glass from a broken beer bottle or the top of a can; Of hop-scotch and 4 squares

❖ Memories of borrowing an egg from a neighbor to complete the corn bread and reciprocating that loan with a cup of sugar to finish off her cake; Of sharing babysitting duties and after school care

❖ Memories of studying the Word of God and praising Him for His Word; Of shouting and dancing all over the sanctuary because you know that God answers prayer

❖ Memories of 'operettas and musicals'; Of church plays and seeing who could remember the longest Easter speech

❖ Memories of laughter after moments of falling tears

❖ Memories of planning family outings and Church picnics; Of dining together at Thanksgiving and sharing at Christmas

❖ Memories of seeing siblings who have moved away from home, but return with hugs and kisses and statements of "I miss you." Of singing around the piano and one person singing off key

❖ Memories of the daughter coming home from college; Of graduations, weddings and grandchildren

❖ Memories of comfort from the man you committed your love to some 58 years ago; Of early morning talks over a cup of coffee with just you and him

❖ Memories of children playing in the backyard and escaping to the front yard where you screamed, "Don't get too close to that street"; Of streetlights and calls from mothers to children to come in because those lights were on

❖ Memories of walking your friend half way home and then she walks you a "piece of the way" back home

❖ Memories of the milk man who drove by and knew your order without asking; Of the mail man that never got your mail confused with the neighbors'

❖ Memories of the corner store with jars of pickles, cookies that were 2 for 1 cent and candy that had money on the inside

❖ Memories of the talent seen on the Ed Sullivan show and witnessing danger on "I Spy!"

❖ Memories of the joy of caring and knowing that someone cares for you!

We have **memories** in the corners of our minds that no one can take away because they are only ours to keep. Ever so often, we see a glimmer of light shining through the countenance of a mind that is far away. A memory is being retrieved of days gone by whose importance was not realized until they became memories. We must learn to cherish our precious moments with family, friends and loved ones, before they become memories. Make a mental note of a pretty smile, a pat on the back, a kiss goodbye so that it will be stored for later use. We must remember. We look at pictures and begin to smile, because we remember. We look at our children and see ourselves, because we remember. We experience a warm feeling inside because we remember. **Thank God for the Memories!**

Our memories of Mama and the life she lived will always be good. Sure there were some tough times; times of not understanding why she said or did what she did as a parent, but I cannot think of a thing that we would change. No matter how dreadful it seemed at the time, we made it through. Our parents provided a caring and safe environment. We were clothed. There was shelter over our heads. We were never hungry.

We were chastised and loved, instructed and punished if we did not adhere to the instructions. My parents were always looking out for our best interests whether we agreed with the plan or not. We were exposed to a better life than the one we were experiencing. We were never limited to what we could do with our own lives. We were told, in other words, to go for it. Dreams were set high. Who could ask for much more than that?

Exposure could very well be the solution to some of the ills of our inner city children today. I am speaking of the children who seem to lack ambition. Sometimes we accept what has been passed down to us because we have never seen anything different. It is a different world. In the movie, Trading Places, one rich character's life is exchanged for the life of a poor street hustler. The point was made that if you change the environment and equalize the playing field, anyone can succeed. Our parents chose to expose us to different ways of life and allowed us to pursue different endeavors even if they never did or could not afford to do so themselves. Memories were made.

The choice was ours. If you received little, it was because you chose little. It was not because they did not offer us the opportunity to choose another path. We took trips: family, school and church sponsored. If you showed some initiative, Mama made the provision with God's help. If you wanted to go to college or trade school, the offer of assistance was extended. If you chose not to, you were on your own. That is a good memory, to know that your parents were behind your endeavors.

What a wonderful thing God did for us when he set up a human computer system that allows us to add, update and delete! Some things need to be permanently destroyed in the trash bin, while some things need to be retrieved. Some things should be placed in 'My Favorites' that is a computer's 'Safe Place'. Only God could have put the significant parts of the brain in place. Our memory, our speech, our thoughts and our emotions all play a vital part in who we are. The evil things can be changed. The evil spirits cast out. What was born can be born again and reborn if necessary.

Miraculous! Memories can be altered to include things that are good. We actually repress unfavorable challenges. The choice is ours. We are guilty of having selective memory. What happens when the choice has been removed? Hopefully, it is at that time our memory basket is filled with mostly good stuff. Only the expressions on Mama's face can indicate what type of memory is being retrieved. The control switch has been altered. The communication system changed, but the memories are the same in a *'Safe Place'*.

CHAPTER II
Mama

Mama was the core of our family. She was the pillar of strength. Her strict, but insightful ways had us questioning if love existed or something was wrong with us. She was so determined that we would be "good" children that often times she went to the extreme with her punishment and chastisement. We never understood why she was so strict. We thought we were very good children. (In the sight of what child is he or she not good?) In later years we found out that this was how she was reared and felt it necessary to bring up her offspring in the same manner. We are all alive today with no prison records, drug overdoses or runaway accounts. Her manner may have been harsh, but it was effective.

God has given instructions in His Holy Word how to rear children. Below are some of those:

Proverbs 13:24 – "He that spareth his rod hateth his son; but he that loveth him chasteneth him quickly."

Proverbs 22:6 – "Train up a child in the way he should go: and when he is old, he will not depart from it."

Proverbs 22:15 – "Foolishness is bound in the heart of a child; but the rod of correction shall drive it far from him."

Ephesians 6:4 – "And, ye fathers, provoke not your children to wrath: but bring them up in the nurture and admonition of the Lord."

This is not child abuse. This is the pattern God set for rearing newly uninformed beings placed on earth; namely children. Wise chastening is not foolish abuse. There is a balance. We are responsible for our offspring. Nurturing, loving, educating and watching over them is our God given duty. We cannot take it lightly. God provided the way. It is our job to understand it and execute it. As he chastises us because He loves us, so must we chastise the ones that we love. We must apply wisdom. What it takes for one child may not be effective with another. Use good judgment and guidance of the Holy Ghost.

Chastisement is not fun, but if we do not implement it the enemy will exercise it, with jailhouse sentences and prison records. I could never understand the statement, "This is going to hurt me more than it is going to hurt you," when I was on the hurting end of the belt. As an adult, with three children of my own, I now understand. It is not a good feeling to spank or even take away privileges from a child, but "No" is an answer that they must learn. If the response is always "Yes," "I believe you," "You did wrong, but it's okay," we will rear a generation of murderers, thieves and rapists. You cannot always say "Yes" to a child. Allow them to experience "No" and some rejection. When they become adults it will not be as difficult to accept. A spoiled child is a rotten adult.

Ephesians 6:1 – "Children obey your parents in the Lord: for this is right. Honor thy father and mother: which is the first commandment with promise." Children do not emerge from the womb reciting this scripture. Neither do they exit the womb with a computer chip ready to be inserted with necessary 'obey your parents' scriptures. Scripture must be taught so that they may understand the way of God. We were taught that obedience was better than a whipping, oh, I mean better than sacrifice. If you did not obey, you sacrificed some part of your body. If only we would obey God, life could be so different. We venture from the path of God, His teachings, commandments and statutes to eventually find out that His way is always the best for our lives. We, like the Israelites, make an 11-day journey to the Promised Land into a 40-year trip through the wilderness because we fail to obey.

Colossians 3:20 – "Children, obey your parents in all things: for this is well pleasing unto the Lord". We learned to desire to please God. When we pleased Him, pleasing Mama came easy. This is a maturing step in life. We grow up trying to please our friends, associates and relatives. If we would strive to please God, all the others would fall in place. **Matthew 6:33** - "But seek ye first the kingdom of God, and his righteousness;

and all these things shall be added unto you." When we seek God first, he will cause everything in our lives to line up; the children, the spouse, the friends, and the boss on the job. We should seek to please Him who has charge over our lives.

A God-fearing Upbringing

Mama taught us all about Jesus. We were practically born and reared in the church. It was all we knew for extra curricular activity. We attended Sunday school, morning worship, Baptist Training Union (even when no one was there, but us, the Kepney children) and night service. We went to musicals, dedicatory programs, mission boards and you name it. Mama was faithful to all of her hats in church. She would spend hours at home figuring out church projects and programs. The church was her heart. She loved the work and was good at it. If someone hurt her feelings, she would pout, fuss with my daddy and then go right back to that church that she had sworn to never set foot in again, and she took our feet with her.

Mama held an office in the citywide conference of churches to which she was extremely dedicated.

Because of this alone, she was well known in many of the area churches. Her speaking engagements were numerous. She built a reputation of being biblically sound and trustworthy. If you placed her name on program, you would not be disappointed and you did not have to worry whether or not she would show up. She was a busy lady, but her family never went lacking. Mama kept up with the church activities and the family ones also. She demonstrated order and organization. We felt her love at all times.

The weekly church routine was something like this: Monday nights - Mission meeting, Tuesday nights - Choir rehearsal, Wednesday nights - Prayer meeting, Saturday - Children's choir rehearsal, Sunday AM - Sunday School, Morning Worship, Afternoon – 2:00pm Communion, Baptist Training Union and Evening - Night Service.

If we are not saved it is not because we did not go to church! If you did not know about God, it was not because you were not in place to learn. There were plenty of legal opportunities to meet the Creator. The household rule was, if you could party or play the night before surely you would not have a problem getting up and going to church (all day) on Sunday. Church was just a part of us.

Though we often complained, it was good for us. When any of us left the household, the Spirit of Worship remained in us. No matter what we did or where we went, Sunday was a designated 'church' day. One of the first things I searched for when I went off to college was a church to go to on Sunday morning. When any of us left home for good there was no question whether we were going to join a local fellowship; the question was which one?

Keep It Holy

Other concrete rules were in place. The Sabbath was to be kept Holy. Among other things, that also meant no shopping on Sunday. My sister, Patricia, failed to secure a pair of stockings one Saturday and had none to wear on Sunday morning to church. She was allowed to stop at the 7 Eleven (this was rare), but it would be the only stop and she would have to wear whatever color or size they had. It just so happened that they were all out of her size and color. All day Sunday Patricia had to suffer with panty hose that she could only pull up midway her thighs and were vanilla in color. Ladies, can you imagine how uncomfortable that must have been? It was our laugh for the day. Just thinking about it kept us awake in church. In fact, I am still laughing!

Individual Assignments

Chores were to be done in absolute perfection. Clothes hung outside on the clothes line had to be uniformed. All shirts together, all underwear together, sheets on the back row and pants hung upside down with the crease in place. We could all work at One Hour Martinizing because if it was one thing we learned how to do and do well, it was how to iron. This was at a time when starch was mixed in the sink and clothes were rolled and placed in the refrigerator until ironing time. Daddy's khaki work pants looked brand new every morning when he left for work. Those pants could stand up on their own. We were taught how to starch dollies and have them stand up. These were placed on the end tables or the back of the sofa. Pillowcases had to be starched, ironed, folded and neatly placed on the shelf. I was so glad when permanent press came on the scene I did not know what to do! She actually expected us to still iron the permanent press! Our rooms had to be in topnotch shape. Even the closets had to exhibit some type of order. She was a neat nick, a trait that she passed on to her daughters. Our homes are kept in such meticulous order that our husbands can never complain.

There was a high level of perfection assigned to each chore. Mama was one of those parents who would let punishments add up. That was the wrong thing to do. When she would finally get to punish you, there was a list of old and new. Once my sister Wilma did not iron a pair of pants that would show a defined crease in the front and back of the pants. I was home for the weekend from college. I had not seen any whipping action in a long time. I felt the heat rising. Mama whipped Wilma not only for the pants, but for the dirty dishes, the closet that was in disarray and everything else she could think of at that time. By the time Wilma finished those pants, they looked brand new!

Even though Mama had strict rules and regulations, they were for our benefit. Our chores freed her hands to cook for us, to clean what we missed and take up where we left off. She had time to pray for us and with us. She had time to study God's Word and keep her household where Jesus could come at anytime to visit. She had time to honor the Prince of the house, my father. She had time to fuss at us, chastise us, and make us angry while continuing to nurture us as her offspring.

Mama woke early in the morning to fix my father's coffee, breakfast and lunch. She worked 40 hours a week and yet my father never had to wonder if he would have any dinner. She made us eat together, pray together and commune with one another. She is a virtuous woman. Her price is far above rubies. Her husband trusted her so that he has no need of spoil. She did him good and not evil all the days of his life. She mended and sewed the clothes of her family. She introduced to us more than the mundane everyday meals by experimenting every now and then with recipes found on the back of boxes or in magazines. She invested the money in items of value that would last and not be easily destroyed. She worked hard on her job and in our home. Mama made sure that we had enough supplies and food. She was compassionate to our neighbors. She was a bold woman and walked unafraid. Strength and honor are her clothing; and she shall rejoice in time to come. She opened her mouth with wisdom and on her tongue was the law of kindness.

Mama looked well to the ways of her household and did not eat the bread of idleness. We rose up and we called her blessed. My father praised her. She excels the greatest of mothers and wives. "Favor is deceitful, and beauty is vain: but a woman that feareth the Lord, she shall be praised. Give her of the fruit of her hands; and let her own works praise her in the gates." *(Proverbs 31:30-31)*. The reverential fear of God exhibited by Mama was as genuine as they come. Her Hallelujah's were forceful and her "Thank You Jesus'" would make you tremble. Her hands were seldom idle. There was plenty work to be done and she was not going to rest until it was completed. It was then and only then at the point of completion would she rest and allow us to rest with her!

CHAPTER III
Bill

William 'Bill' Kepney was the love of Mama's life. Married on December 23, 1945, the two were inseparable until death. She was the beautiful young thing that captured his heart. He was the slim young man that worked at the garage and came to the diner for lunch where she worked. She listened for his whistles as he turned the corner coming through the alley to get to her diner. Whether it was for the sandwich or the glimpse of Leona, it was a daily trip that he looked forward to taking and she looked forward to his coming. Leona was the first one to call him Bill. William called her Lee. He cherished her. She adored him. There was nothing that was beyond his reach that he would not do for her. They shared everything: friends, family, jokes and yes, their belief in God. It led to a lustrous love affair that lasted through 7 children (3 deceased), 2 houses, 13 dogs and over 58 years.

God and communication in a marriage is the key to a long, enduring relationship. Early morning talks over a cup of coffee consisted of the previous day's experiences with the 'children', the church and the upcoming events for the day. It was a peaceful time when most of the family members were still asleep. They would even let the dog in to the kitchen for a little quiet time. These were precious moments to them that took place about 5:30am every morning without fail. She would get up and fix his lunch before he left for work and they would take the time to chat before they started the day. Even though most of the time we were fast asleep, they would invite us into these chats if you just happened to wake up and get up out of bed that early in the morning.

The ways of the household were 'Bill' centered. We ate dinner when Bill came home from work. He said the grace. The turkey was carved by him and him only on holidays. Sometimes, chastisement was on hold until he came home. You would often hear, "Wait until your daddy comes home." We really preferred his chastening because it was shorter. He would give you a few licks and was done. You cried a little and then went outside to play. Daddy was afraid of hurting us. Mama, on the other hand, did not know when enough was enough. We would spend one third of the time running and she spent one third of the time trying to catch us. The rest was history.

Daddy was the sportsman and game player in the family. Sports and games were not Mama's cup of tea. This was one area that they complemented each other. He played games and played all the time. She let him know just how far he could go with his playing. Daddy loved to play games. He loved cards, dominoes (which he taught me – I learned from the best), and bowling. Nothing was too elementary for him to play to bond with his children. Daddy played jacks, pick up sticks, badminton, four squares, etc. That spirit carried over into our own families. If you fellowship with the

Kepney clan there are three things you are bound to do: go to church, eat and play games.

Fishing was Daddy's get away; his quiet time. He lived to fish. He would be gone all day on Saturdays fishing. Toledo Bend, Louisiana was his favorite spot. He would fish from the shore and sometimes in a boat if he could rent one. He would bring the fish home, clean it and if Mama did not want to be bothered, he would give it to the neighbors. He tried to make us interested in fishing, but it did not go over too well. We just did not share the love of fishing, but we do however, love the water.

Another talent that he seemed to have passed on to his children was his ability to sing. Daddy had a lovely velvety voice that could have been marketed. He sang in the church choir and sometimes did solos when I was a child. As a deacon, he was given the privilege of 'raising a hymn' every now and then. His voice would seem to resonate throughout the building and even if you were on the outside, and could hear, you knew it was Deacon Kepney singing. He always wanted us to display our gifts as well. He encouraged my brother Darrell to sing because he sang with such spirit. My sister, Patricia, has an awesome singing range, but is shy about her gift. Wilma and I are the alto/tenors that were always teased because of our low voices. Mama could also sing and as they did everything else, it was rare, but wonderful when she and Daddy sang together.

A peaceful household was of utmost importance with our father. I firmly believe that the 'peace' DNA we received came from him. He would go to the extreme to keep peace. Whatever it took to make everybody happy, he felt was his job to accomplish. I had a kindergarten teacher that insisted on my eating oatmeal for breakfast. I hated oatmeal. My mother was all for executing this ritual because it was a good nutritional idea. Whenever possible she would cook oatmeal for breakfast. To make up for the unpleasant breakfast consumed the day before, my daddy would quietly ask me what I wanted for breakfast for the next day. My respond would be pork chops and French fries. He would get up early enough to fix it and I would enjoy. We would wait until Mama had left for work. It was our secret. It did not kill me!

We were taught to respect our father regardless of what he said or did. We never heard a negative word against him. The love that Mama had for him, was imputed to us and we accepted it. Mama was very grateful for the name my father gave her. In 1995 she attended a Women's Conference in St Louis, Missouri, where I was the keynote speaker. I was introduced as Evangelist Gladys White. My mother kindly corrected the Mistress of Ceremony by saying, "That is Gladys Kepney White." At the banquet table she reminded me that I was a Kepney first and would always be one. She had taken on that name and it was the last name of all of her children. It was important to her never to forget who you were and from whence you came. As a tribute to her, I never leave off the Kepney in my name.

My Daddy was an extraordinary man. (I say My Daddy because that is what I called him for the 11 beautiful years that I was an only child. He informed me that I had to share; he was not only my daddy, but daddy to the other three people they brought into the house from the hospital.) My Daddy loved God, his wife and his children. He loved life. He worked hard to provide for his family. He gave the company that he worked for over 30 years of service. He served large party engagements as a side job. He would bring home some samples of the rich delicacies that were served. We would eagerly await his arrival to see what he would bring that we had never tasted before.

There were never any serious needs or desires suffered in our house. If there were, the children never knew it. The provision we experienced as children continued through adulthood. If he thought we were in need of anything his question was: "Baby, How can daddy help?" We had this family pact that we would send each other birthday money that was equivalent to our age. If you were 39 you received $39 from each family member. When it was the next person's birthday you had to send money equivalent to their age. If Daddy had received all of his money, he would have always come out on top. Unfortunately, there was always someone coming up short. Some of whom owe me now. I called him one year to explain that my money was funny, but I would send his birthday gift/money on my next payday. He wired me a hundred dollars on his birthday. That was the type father he was – always providing.

Mama taught us girls the importance of submitting to a good man. Submission is easier (not impossible, but easier) when you have been blessed with a good god-fearing man. My daddy was a prime example of that kind of man. We are all independent, very outspoken women, but we know just how far we can go with our own husbands. There is a statute of limitation. Daddy would never hit my mother, but she also knew just how far she could push him before she hit the wrong button. Arguments would get heated, with Mama doing all of the fussing. She pretty much wanted things her way and he allowed it for as long as he could stand it. He would always say "Check with your Mama" or "Well, you know your Mama." He knew her well and respected her decisions for the family.

Our parents' marital goal was to please God and each other. Every birthday and anniversary was celebrated. No gift was too extravagant; no distance too far. They shared friends, desires, dreams, hopes, family, coffee and a love for God. They were inseparable. They were best friends who never wished to leave each other, but included each other in all endeavors. Major decisions were laid out on the kitchen table and discussed. An agreement was made and carried through. Many board meetings were held at that kitchen table; many laws passed regarding the children and the household, many trips decided, many fund raisers discussed and many meals planned.

When things began to happen to Mama, Daddy initially chose not to understand, but eventually he accepted what had to be done. The love never ended. He would visit her daily. He would talk with her about things that were going on, how the children were doing and how the church was progressing. It was a difficult task, but he endured it without complaint. He told us repeatedly the hardest thing he had to do was to leave her in the nursing home. She would say, "Bill, please don't leave me." Not knowing whether she really recognized him or not, it would still crush his spirits to leave her.

Love covers a multitude of faults. They were not perfect and neither was their marriage, but it lasted over five decades. It was a love of real commitment that expressed a feeling of no matter what you do, I love you. Nothing and nobody can change that. They had their heated discussions and falling outs, but they managed to always mend the broken pieces and correct the misunderstandings. There was never any talk of separation (that the children heard). They supported each other as though no one else would and they taught us to support each other as well. If you talked about one Kepney, you talked about and had to face the whole clan.

The love shared between the two of them should have been witnessed by the world. It was a love that had no end. Even death could not end it. She does not know 'not to love him'. He never knew not to love her. He would tell us that he did not quite understand why this happened to her, but he still loved her. The peace she had when she last saw him remains and so does the love. Funny thing – God spared her the separation and pain of his demise. She has memories of him that are yet alive in her mind when she chooses to bring them up.

When Daddy left and went home to live with God, we were not ready. We had no idea that this would happen. We knew that he was on medication for his thyroid condition, but never expected him to leave when he did. We tried to explain to Mama that he was gone, but it never registered. I guess we are glad about that. She will always have memories of him alive and well. She will remember his love and constant protection of his family. Perhaps she would someday remember how much he loved her and his children. Hopefully, she will remember what a good provider he was. She will remember that he was a strong, but a gentle man. She will remember his big smile and haughty laughter. She can cherish those memories, whenever they come up. Perhaps some of her misunderstood smiles are memories of a love that surpassed our understanding that we can only wish for ourselves.

My Daddy, we miss you so very much!

CHAPTER IV
The Children

It would be ideal to state that from the union of William and Leona came four of the most well adjusted, successful, law abiding citizens that ever were reared in the United States of America. It could be said. It just would not be the truth. The Kepney offspring were average children and typical teenagers. I am sure we caused as much heartache as any of the other kids on the block. We were adventurous babies, rambunctious tots, flip mouth pre-teens and know-it-all, but do not know anything teens. In spite of the strict upbringing, we still acted and talked like children and when of age behaved like Western teens.

Mama loved her children. Regardless of our faults and failures, she loved us. She bragged on us and insulted us in the same breath. She secretly thanked God for us (I know this because I heard her talking to someone on the phone). The cruel and unusual punishment (the way we saw it as children) was her way of bending the sap. She was so determined that we would be 'good' children that her methods were often times intense. The Bible states who God loves, He chastises. Trust me, there was plenty of love at our address. As painful as it was to our backsides and our feelings, it did not destroy us. Instead, it did instill character in us all.

The tables have turned. No longer are the people who were taking care of all of our business and handling our affairs, whether we liked it or not, doing that any more, but instead we are handling theirs. Remember when you were young and you could not wait to be 'grown'? You made stupid statements like, "I cannot wait to leave this house" not knowing that this included working, buying gas, paying rent, buying groceries and paying utility bills. How about the statement, "When I have children I am not going to..." Now you wish your parents would rear yours. You see the same characteristics in your children that were in you. They make the same mistakes. Their response to your judgment is predictable. You know all of the answers. You begin to gradually understand the purpose of chastisement and the word 'No'. You find yourself dishing out some of the same advice and punishments that you swore as a child you would not use against your own children.

Did you ever say, "Mama, you just don't understand; it's different today than it was in your day?" Now you live with some young person who thinks he or she knows everything and you are the old foggy that is in the dark. They swear things are different now then when you were growing up. In my studies of life, I have found that life is a circle. What goes around eventually comes back around. Fads, hairstyles, clothing styles all fade out, but eventually return to the forefront. It is possible to keep clothes for 10 to 15 years and they will in due course come back in style. Young people are convinced that we adults are in the dark with no light ever to be shown. What they do not know is that we really have done that and we actually have been there before!

The Kepney Children were no different than any other children. We wanted so badly to leave what we thought was temporary incarceration. We did not know how good we had it. We had two loving parents in the house. Some of our friends were products of broken homes or single parents. We had two who looked out for not only our present well being, but also our futures. Somebody else was concerned about making ends meet. Someone else was praying for the words to say to get through to their children. All we could perceive were two old folks who did not understand today's kids and what we were going through. When they would make statements like, "I have been where you are going" we would say, "Yeah, right." Boy, were we clueless.

When we were separated from our parents we experimented with everything possible. Whenever it was something against what was drilled in us, we could always hear that soprano voice say, "Didn't I tell you not to do that, you better not do that!" We looked and Mama was not around, but she was definitely heard. You see, we were brought up in a time in which fear played a great part in bringing up a child. The general consensus was that if the fear of the parent was prevalent, crimes committed were at a minimum. This was a reverential fear. It was not a fear for our lives, but a respect for the authority that fed you, clothed you and provided shelter for you. Restrictions were in place and we had to abide by them.

All of my siblings live in a different state than I do. We have made an unwritten rule that we will not let three months go by without talking to each other. In fact, we make weekly contact. We were taught to watch out for each other. It was by example that we learned to love not hate, be jealous of or envious of one another. Hatred is a learned emotion; it has to be taught. It was not even mentioned in the Kepney household. Prejudice was not allowed. Our parents were not partial towards us and we were not towards each other. Jealousy and envy were never welcomed. If Mama brought Darrell something home, the girls would not dare ask where is mine. We just waited our turn. Negative emotions need to be addressed at the onset. When they are left to fester, gigantic problems can occur. If you live in peace at home, chances are you can do the same outside of the home. *Hebrews 12:9* came easy, "Follow peace with all men..."

The Kepney children share a wonderful bond. We can feel each other's cares. We pray for our Mother and each other. When a nephew or niece is in trouble, we pitch in to see what we can do as a family. Oh yeah, we argue, but we agree to disagree. Our father believed in tranquility. He would allow Mama to fuss, scream and holler, but he would remain calm until she finished and then let her have her way. He knew about a woman's fury and he realized when he was in a no-win situation. That same quality was passed on to my brother Darrell. He loves peace. If one sister fell out with another, Darrell was the go-between; the mediator to mend the relationship. He is the peacemaker of the family.

We believe and support one another. Milestones are awarded. If any family member was performing somewhere, as many as could, would get there to support. On several occasions, I had the blessed opportunity to preach in Houston. My sister, Patricia, would call up all of our relatives in the Houston area, make the announcement of when and where I would be preaching and would expect them to be there. It was always like a mini reunion. After the occasion expired, we would all dine together at a local restaurant. There is nothing like family support. Our children are included in that support. Graduations, baptisms, weddings, even funerals of in-laws, plays, etc are attended whether it is your child, a nephew or a niece. It is called 'love'.

Love with a Smile

Laughter is so good for the human spirit. It is a type of healer. When the Kepney children get together, we laugh. From the moment we see each other until the last person leaves, we laugh. We have invited friends from our various environments and had them to taste the Kepney humor. No one has left us untouched by the laughter we share. Laughter can be a means of coping although balance has to be determined. Too much laughter and you might go over the edge, but in its proper place and quantity it is good for us. When you can see the humor in a situation that seems so dreadful, you can better receive the consequences. When the human spirit is at peace, then decision-making is profitable. If our minds and hearts are wrapped in a bad situation and there is no peace our answers may not work for our good. I thank God for laughter. He has given a release other than our tears.

We are a family of many talents. We provide opportunities to showcase our gifts among each other. It is imperative that you study to show yourself approved. If you have not perfected that talent, there is the possibility of receiving ridicule (in fun). If you come, you got to come right! We have Apollo Night (a type of talent show). We are competitive. We play games with each other and our children. When we dine together, everybody is responsible for a particular dish. It comes together. No one person has to do it all. We share the responsibility of the event just as we share the responsibility of Mama. No one is left out. We are a family! It is called: 'love'.

We are such a blessed family. We had a great start. It is up to us, the Kepney children, to keep what was started in 1945 going. Every family member should look at his or her family as a personal responsibility. If I fail to do my part I injure the structure. If one falls, I am responsible for his or her recovery. That is what family is all about. Because we are familiar, meaning we have the same genes, the same ancestors, the same upbringing, the same parents, and generally reared in the same environment, we are family.

God instituted the family unit long before He put the 'church' in place. He makes us understand how important our family is throughout the Bible. This prepares us to become good citizens in His kingdom. Selfish motives have to be replaced with consideration of another. Once we grasp the significance of the family and how it is the representation of one, then we are ready to be a part of the greatest family of all – the Body of Christ.

CHAPTER V
THE CHURCH

Now, let us talk about the church. Mama's name should be right next to the definition of the word 'church' in the dictionary as a synonym. She believed strongly in the power of prayer and church fellowship. The church is an institution established in the Kingdom Age by Christ himself when He spoke to Peter in *Matthew 16* and said "...and upon this rock I will build my church; and the gates of hell shall not prevail against it." That scripture was reiterated constantly in the Kepney household from the moment the marriage vows were spoken. The church is a body of baptized believers. Most of us were baptized early in our family; pretty much right after we learned to read and could tell the preacher, "yes" when he asked, "Do you believe in God?"

The church was a priority in our house. Everyone was expected to go to church. We have always known that it was God's will that we attend church. "Not forsaking the assembling of ourselves together as the manner of some is; but exhorting one another: and so much the more, as ye see the day approaching." (*Hebrews 10:25*) Both good and bad habits are formed in a life time. Church was a good habit that was not easily broken. We were going to church on Sunday even if we stayed out until the wee hours of the morning or until the sun rose on that Sunday morning. The commandment was: if you can party; you can go to church. If attendance could save you, we would be a 'sure in'!

Keeping things in righteous perspective, Mama took care of the things of the household Monday through Saturday, but on Sunday morning she got up with her sights set on getting to church. As much work, as possible, was completed on Saturday. Daddy's handkerchiefs were ironed, and we had a pretty good idea what we were expected to wear. Mama would start cooking breakfast at about 6:00am that Sunday morning, (most of the time dinner as well). She would then call us to the table to eat, command the clean up and rush us out of the house for 9 o'clock Sunday school.

We kept the day Holy. We were at church at least 9 hours of the day. It was so instilled in us that when I would come home for the weekend from college, my siblings and I would search for churches that were having musicals, solo hours or gospel concerts; just some kind of church. Church was all we knew. During a family reunion in Houston when all of the activities had come to a halt, the young people gathered to discuss what we would do that Saturday night. We had cousins from Texas, Louisiana, Missouri and me from Alabama. We were from the ages of about 22 to 35 or so. Our cousins were naming 'hot spots' that they had heard were in Houston; places where they could dance and get their drink 'on'. The Kepney's were suggesting the movies or a game night at my sister's house. One of my cousins commented, "We did not come to Houston to go to the movies, we can do that at home." Well, the Kepneys did not know how to 'club' or we had gotten past that stage of our lives. All we knew was church! Consequently, our little close-knit group went to Blockbuster Video, picked up some movies and went to my sister's house for our entertainment. We were just fine with being together.

At our 1985 family reunion, held in St Louis, MO, as we were deciding where the 1987 reunion would be held, the volunteer for the future festivities came from the California relatives. My aunt outlined the activities of what she thought would be a grand family affair: a Get Acquainted Night, a Picnic, a tour of Los Angeles, a Family Banquet and some free time. She left an opening for suggestions. We noticed that there was no mention of when or where the family would worship together. There was no 'church' in her itinerary. Has she got the right family? She was immediately bombarded with the question, "When do we go to church?" My aunt, who is ever so eloquent, stated, "We can find a church to go to, if you like." We graciously explained to her that most of us were from the Deep South, and that is what we do - we go to church; saints and sinners alike!

An old cliché states that a family that prays together stays together. I submit that a family that attends church together and believes God's Word stays together as well. It is true. When God is first in anything we do, the glue factor is there. He becomes that element that keeps us together. Families must endure good times as well as hard times together. When you do not have anybody else, you have your family. People who have been adopted occasionally have a feeling of loneliness. They will search diligently for relatives just to feel that sense of family; that sense of belonging. As previously stated, the church is a body of baptized believers from various households. These believers commonly accept the same doctrine and explanation of truth. The church body is a family made up of different families. Therefore, what was prevalent in our home was an assurance that outside of our immediate family, we had an extended family in the church.

Never were we to feel that we were alone. Solace was in the church. If the answer was not in the parent, we could go to the church. The church represented not just the edifice where praise, worship, prayers and a sermon took place, but a place inside of us where the Spirit of God abided. Praise and worship is a personal experience that does not need a certain number of people or a certain place to be exercised. The building is where the body of Christ, the family of believers comes to worship. The edifice shelters the 'church body' (the people who make up the church) in one place. Hopefully the body is on one accord. The fact remains that the true church is in us! We bring the church to the building.

The church represented a place of contentment. Getting involved with the things that cause the church to thrive left less time to worry about personal issues or get into trouble. Church ministries, then known as auxiliaries, were plentiful. There was always something going on that would captivate your interest and utilize your talent. The choir was for those who love to sing, the usher board for those who love to serve, Sunday school for learning, youth activities for the young people to get involved. These things could keep you out of trouble, and also allowed you to realize through sharing that you are not in any boat alone.

The enemy's tactic has always been to divide and conquer. He knows that if he can get one individual to a point of anger or disappointment in the fellowship, he can manipulate others to his plan. That is why he attacks our personal 'church'. He wants to destroy the family so he starts with just one person. After he has secured the one, he goes after the group. The enemy divides us in doctrine. Just the word 'denomination' denotes division. In the Gospel according to Matthew, Christ established only one church. We are the ones who brought about the division. We allow the enemy to divide us in what we believe. It is strange how we all use the same Bible, but we end up with thousands of interpretations of doctrine. Never give place to the enemy. Never let him see you sweat. Speak togetherness of the churches and not division. He wants us divided and in rare cases we are, but he has never read the end of the story: the church still prevails!

Galatians 5:20 speaks against seditions. This is rebellion with an argumentative spirit; designed to separate and destroy. We have to be careful not to be used of the enemy. He creeps into our 'church' with adultery, fornication, uncleanness, lasciviousness, idolatry, witchcraft, variance, emulations, wrath, strife, seditions, heresies, envyings, murders, drunkenness, revellings, jealousy, slothfulness, murmuring and complaining. These spirits will cause division in the church body. They devastate lives, break up homes and split churches. The church has to be mindful of the inward building that has been swept and garnished. If evil spirits are not replaced by that of the Holy Ghost, according to *Matthew 12:44,* one evil spirit will return with seven more.

On a more personal level, once we have been cleaned and have changed our minds against sin and our hearts toward God, we have to replace that vacant territory with the Holy Ghost. Mama loved to say, "An idle mind is the devil's workshop." This statement was simple, but profound. The Word of God encourages us to pray without ceasing, study to show ourselves approved, meditate on the Word day and night, become holy and to present our bodies as a living sacrifice all in an effort to keep us saved. The drinking, the smoking, the adultery, the fornication or whatever the sin or weight may be that God has freed you from, has to be replaced with something else. Replace your evil with good. Get involved with Kingdom work. If you allow the enemy a lazy moment he will take advantage of it. Give the devil no place and no opportunity!

We have the blessed assurance that the gates of hell will not prevail against the church. We are the church and God has established it. Weapons may form against it, but they shall not prosper. We were taught to believe in the church because it will stand forever!

CHAPTER VI
Beliefs

Everything has a beginning; even this earth. In the beginning there was God. Most Christians believe and accept that nothing existed before there was God. The world was without form and void. God is the creator of the universe and all that is in it; including mankind. He is Alpha and Omega. He is the beginning and He is the end. God is the Great I Am. He said unto Moses, "I AM THAT I AM." He is everything you need him to be. He is the King of kings and the Lord of lords. God is a strong tower. He is our refuge. He is someone we can trust. Without Him nothing is and nothing can be. He is and was and forever will be. You cannot add to Him and you cannot take away from Him. God is absolute. God just 'is'.

If all Christians are in agreement with the aforementioned attributes of God, the enemy should be on the run. Christ said in *John 14:12,*"Greater works shall ye do." This word 'greater' denotes more good works. In this dispensation of time, we have more means of communication to reach people with the good news of the gospel. We have cable television, radio, satellite, postal mail, E-mail, and the like. We have faster travel accommodations. Jesus and the disciples traveled on foot. We have been invested with much greater power and resources! Because of modern technology alone, we should be doing more than the disciples ever dreamed of doing. Books are written to explain the Word of God, songs are composed to inspire us through the Word of God, and even the media has to announce the truths and power of God when unexplainable events occur.

God's power is noticeable in the seasons. Seasons come and seasons go. Certain catastrophes are common in certain areas: tornadoes in the central states, hurricanes in the south, winter blizzards in the north and earthquakes in the western states. It is His power that acts as a catalyst to man's ingenuity. God has been so kind to allow man to determine when these storms will occur and how to deal with them yet leaving an element of surprise with each one that we may continue to look to Him for safety.

God intervenes with miracles that occur in our lives daily: organ transplants, Siamese twin separations, cancer cures, space walks, and electronic inventions. God's power is inexhaustible and He is so good that He shares it with us; He does not share His glory, but His power. He gives us the ability to fight back the elements when they are out of control, to heal our bodies when they have been invaded with sickness, to make new discoveries here on earth and in space and to make amazing gadgets that enhance our lives.

Mama experienced that 'power' of God. She is a woman who knew God intimately! She had close encounters of a God kind; a personal relationship with her Heavenly Father. However it was experienced, she shared her God encounters with her family. She knew

God as Savior and as Lord. In Him she moved and had her being. She trusted Him when the money was low and when there was an overflow. She praised Him at both times. Mama agreed that there were two times to praise God: 1) when you feel like it and 2) when you don't. She knew that she could do nothing without Him because without Him she was nothing. She understood His power, felt his presence and trusted Him to know all about her needs in any situation. He was her deliverer from all unpleasant circumstances; a present help in the time of trouble. He was her salvation.

Mama was a busy lady. She was a spiritual educator. Mama taught that in the beginning was the Word and the Word was with God and the Word was God. She taught the Bible from Genesis to Revelation. Throughout the city of Shreveport, she spoke about God at various churches as a Sunday School Superintendent or teacher, Women's Day Speaker or Conference Speaker. She worked at her local church as the Christian Education chairperson, secretary, choir member, Baptist Training Union leader and church maid when necessary. Mama was affiliated with the 13th District Baptist Association (a conglomerate of churches throughout the city). With all this, she was still able to keep watch over her own household and keep the enemy at bay. As a family we lacked nothing. Mama did her works in excellence, with humility and without complaint. She did the 'more' that God said we would do.

We thank God for our mother, Mrs. Leona (Owens) Kepney, a woman of integrity and strong belief in the only Power that 'be'. This same belief was imparted into four children who have passed it on to their children – and the name of God goes on. These children will pass it on to their children and there will be generations of children that are believers in God. A legacy was formed. Houses and land make for a good heritage. Bank trusts, CD's and insurance policies should be passed down to our offspring. All these things could and should be in the plans of a parent when contemplating the future of their children, but all these things can be lost or squandered away. The name of God will last forever. When you have given a child the firm foundation of a life with Jesus Christ you have given him more than money can buy. The consensus at 4914 Dandridge

Place was that it was a house where God's name was perpetual. It was a name of rich inheritance to be carried down from generation to generation.

God instructed Moses in Exodus to tell the children of Israel to continually remind their children of what He did for them when He brought them out of the land of bondage. This was not to be forgotten or taken lightly. My mother would never let us forget where our blessings came from. We thanked God first and for everything. We did not eat before we prayed and we did not sleep until we recognized the God who helped us make it through the day. Her praise was vigorous and it was aggressive! Her worship was sincere. She praised him with her lips, her life, her heart and her finances. Mama loved God with all her strength. She was not embarrassed or ashamed of expressing her gratitude to her God. All Glory was to Him, the giver and sustainer of life!

Waver Not

Mama stood firm in her beliefs. She did not waver. Some of her beliefs were very traditional, because she did not stray far from the old path. There was no working on Sunday. "Six days shall thou labor and do all thou work; But, the seventh day is the Sabbath of the Lord thy God: in it thou shalt not do any work, thou, nor thy son, nor thy daughter, thy manservant, nor thy maidservant, nor thy cattle, nor thy stranger that is within thy gate. For in the six days the Lord made heaven and earth, the sea, and all that in them is, and rested the seventh day: wherefore the Lord blessed the Sabbath day, and hallowed it." (*Exodus 20:9-11*)

No ironing, or cleaning took place on Sunday. If you did not iron it on Saturday night, you wore it roughdry on Sunday to church (because you were going to church regardless). If your stockings were not purchased on Saturday, on Sunday you had to wear hosiery with runs in them or a pair that was so short that they had to be held up by a safety pin and prayer. It was of your best interest to prepare for Sunday morning. You were not given many opportunities to make up for not preparing. If you did not prepare, your fate and attire was up to Mama. Not many teens care for their mother choosing their Sunday outfit. God and Mama said no work and that was the end of that!

By whatever means necessary, my mother brought up God-fearing children (and Mama-fearing children). Basic principles were taught and enforced. Morals were high on the agenda. Truth was very important to her. During strict chastisement, you lessened the stripes if you told the truth. Mind you, you were going to be punished, but at least it would not last as long if you told the truth. On the other hand, if you chose not to tell the truth, you prolonged the agony. Whatever you do, do not, and I repeat, do not change your story in the middle of the stream! The risk and the consequences are not worth it.

Mama made 'believers' out of us!

CHAPTER VII
Standards

Every household is governed by rules, whether written or unwritten, set by the leaders of the pact. Certain guide lines are established so that peace and harmony can flow amongst the inhabitants. Chores are assigned and expected to be implemented in a timely manner. Without this form of government the family institution will suffer or even possibly fall apart. If everyone is dutiful to their assignment, there is peace in the valley. Mama laid down the rules and we obeyed them.

Cleanliness was a priority. Even though it is not scriptural, we heard numerous times "Cleanliness is next to Godliness." Personally, I do not think God has a problem with our being clean, but He was surely credited with this statement. We were raised in a house that was just that 'clean'. Chores were individually assigned to keep the house in a 'board of health' condition. You could see yourself in the floors that were mopped, waxed and buffed. The kitchen had to be spotless, before any cooking was started (and we did want to eat). The house had four human dishwashers who could not fight over whose turn it was to do the dishes. Clothes were in their proper place in a neat organized closet. Sheets and pillowcases were starched, ironed to perfection and kept in the hall open-faced closet. When passing by you could see the creases and smell the starch. The bathroom was kept in shining condition. Coming home from college to that bathroom was a pleasure. It was always shiny clean. Dusty furniture was not allowed. Furniture polish was purchased like loaves of bread. Venetian blinds were cleaned blind by blind; always in white glove test condition. Everything was dusted, washed, buffed or polished.

Allowance was considered a part of the household budget, but it was made clear that you were not paid for the chores you worked. This was just a part of the scheme of things. Chores were a way of life. They prepared you for the adult life ahead. Your pay was a good night sleep in a bed in your room and three meals daily. The fact that you got to live there was pay enough. The allowance was so that you could learn the responsibility of handling money and pay for some of the things you were bugging them to purchase for you. We were not reared with the notion that our parents owed us something. We learned to appreciate the many wonderful things they did for us expecting nothing in return.

We were taught to give God his first. Tithing was a part of our learning. Early instructions on tithing helped to make the transition of giving as adults easier. We always knew to tithe. God's 10% was means to a blessing. It belongs to Him. Later in life we knew to look to God as our source. He has, as He promised in his Word, rebuked the devourer on our behalf.

Responsibilities were issued. We had two working parents. Mama came home from working as a school cafeteria manager from 6:00am to 3:00pm, cooked dinner and had it on the table when Daddy came home from work at about 6:30pm every evening. She would allow us to cook occasionally, but she told me one time that if Daddy wanted me to cook, he would have married me. Did not quite make sense to me then, but I got the picture. When of age everyone had to pull his or her own weight.

Responsibility was a great issue in our household. One summer I worked at the same company where my father was a garage attendant. We had to be at work at the same time each morning and got off at the same time each day. I had to pay him $5 a week for gas. Gas then was about 44 cents a gallon, so that $5 nearly filled his vehicle to the brim. I fussed about it, but it taught me responsibility. When I could not find a job during the summer, I had to work as a volunteer at a day care. If a Kepney was of age and did not work, he/she did not eat!

Self-respect and **self worth** were empowered. There was a Kepney standard and we all had to live up to it. No one was exempt. Embarrassing the Kepney name was out of the question. There were things you did not say and places you did not go. You were a representative of the Kepney household and an ambassador for God. Governmental handouts were a no, no! We worked; we earned. We were taught to be independent. No one owed you anything. If there is something you wanted, you had to work for it. You could even convince Mama to pay you for some particular jobs around the house if you did them well.

Being **trustworthy** was strictly enforced. Mama's favorite cliché was, "A man's word is his bond." Mama felt that if you agreed to do something, you must do everything in your power to keep your word. Without your word, you are nothing. Character was judged. You were expected to be trustworthy. There was no calling home to see if you were in place or had completed your chores. Orders were given early and expected to be carried out without fail or reminders.

Mama had to be able to trust you. The bond of trust is easily broken, but very difficult to repair. God trusted

Adam and Eve in the Garden of Eden. Even though God has since allowed man to be reconciled to Him, no one has entered into the Garden of Eden since that fall of man. At the east of the garden, God placed Cherubims and a flaming sword, which turned every way to keep the way of the tree of life. (*Genesis 3:24*) This was to make sure that Adam and Eve did not return. With Mama you started out with so many trust chips, when you exhausted them you left that bosom of trust and it was 'over for you', never to be regained. Freedom lied in her ability to trust us. No trust – no games, no phones, no dates, no freedom, no life.

Education was charged. School was like church – mandatory. It was preparation for a better life. Parents went to PTA, and children went to school. Close contact was established with the teachers and the principals. You were expected to restrain yourself and "act like you had some sense." Suspension was unheard of unless you decided to be suspended from the ceiling. Unlike parents today, Mama would always take the side of the teacher or the adult in charge. You had very little say so, and if an adult had declared you in the wrong, the word of the adult was gospel. You got double for your trouble. There was the possibility of punishment at the school and a repeat performance at home. Parent school visits were for parties, PTA, and rides home in the rain, not because you were in any kind of trouble.

Respect for elders was a must. We said "yes, ma'm" and "no, ma'm"; "yes, sir" and "no, sir". We did not dip into grown folk's conversations. We knew our place and stayed in it. Children were to be seen and not heard. They were excused from the presence of adult conversation. Butting in? There was no such thing! Even an occasional "excuse me" would not suffice. If you got that look of, "boy you better get away from here," then that is what you did and asked your question later. Children ate at the card table until we were invited as adults to sit at the big table. Mama's friends were just that, her friends. She called them by their first name; we had to address them with a "handle": Mr., Mrs. or Miss. Children were children; not little people treated as adults!

Family Unity was stressed and exercised. We were a family in every sense of the word. We went to church together, played together, ate at home and ate out together. We have even taken trips together after becoming adults since we had left the household. The Christmas gathering was rotated among cities: one year in Shreveport, the next year in Mobile and the next in Houston. One year it was too difficult for every one to have the usual Christmas holidays off (plus money was tight) so we had Christmas in March. We exchanged gifts and pretended the tree was up. Every year we exchanged names and laughed at trinkets received. Mama loved giving trinkets.

Pride had its place. We lived in a good neighborhood. Nothing fancy, just good brick houses that a lot of our school cohorts did not have. We were never taught that we were any better than anyone else, but we were made to appreciate what had been done for us and what was given to us. We had hard working parents that provided for us. Whether it was the latest fashion statement or not you were clothed. Current fashion was allowed, but not to be pushed over the rim. Steak and potatoes was not a common meal, but you were fed. The cars under the car port were not Cadillacs or Jaguars, but transportation was provided. Everything had a limit. There was no keeping up with the Jones'. We had ours. They had theirs. A standard was established when it came to our dress attire. Models wore the mini skirts, but the Kepney girls did not. That was kept in the magazine or on TV.

Restrictions

In Mama's house there were restrictions. Her rules of government were consistent. She did not bend. From the oldest to the youngest, the rules were enforced. Just like the Bible, the commandments never changed. If it was sin last year; it is sin this year. Her rules lined up with the Word of God and her punishment was not very short from it, either. The worst thing you could do was to allow the past sins to pile up on you. Mama would let you get by on a few things until that final straw that broke the camel's back. When punishment came, it was for old and new. Your best bet was to get the punishment at time of the crime. There was no statute of limitation. If it came to her memory she added to the corporal punishment. Something you may have forgotten that you had done, Mama remembered.

God set Adam in a place that was both fruitful and beautiful: the Garden of Eden. Adam did not have to toil nor sweat. Everything was provided, but God gave him restrictions. In life there are many restrictions. We are limited as to what we can do and say and remain God-fearing people. *Genesis 2:15-17* states "And the Lord God took the man, and put him into the Garden of Eden to dress it and to keep it. And the Lord God commanded the man, saying, of every tree of the garden thou mayest freely eat: but of the tree of the knowledge of good and evil, thou shalt not eat of it: for in the day that thou eatest thereof thou shalt surely die." Adam ate. Adam ignored the restriction. As God promised, he died. He did not die physically, but he died spiritually because his sin separated him from the Father. A father/son relationship was severed. Restrictions have their place in every Christian household. Without government, chaos abides. Where there is chaos there is no peace. Where there is no peace there is no God.

There are many restrictions in our secular lives as well. We have to respect rules of government because they put us all on the same playing field. The 55mph speeding limit is not just for the Kia, but it is also for the Excursion. So, if you hit me with the Kia or hit me with the Excursion, the insurance will report that the car was damaged by another vehicle and my deductible is the same when hit by either car. Chances are that my policy will be terminated or premium increased. Rules are for the Jew, the Greek and the Gentile. Without rules of government every man would look to himself for justice. God requires us to keep the rules that He set and look to him for righteousness avoiding our own self-righteousness.

Restrictions kept us from abusing and over exercising our rights. When you are a part of a family you have inevitable rights by the mere fact that you are a member. These rights can be abused if you are not careful. When we are born again we become the righteousness of God by the blood that Jesus shed for us on the cross. This gives us some rights and privileges, but it also gives us responsibilities. In *Romans 6:1-2*, Paul warns us regarding the liberty that we have in Christ, "What shall we say then? Shall we continue in sin, that grace may abound? God forbid. How shall we that are dead to sin, live any longer therein?" As responsible Christians we cannot ignore the restrictions that are placed on Holy living. We have to ask ourselves in any given situation, though I can do it, is it right for me to do it?

Love was everywhere. Love was in the home-cooked four-course meals that we received everyday. Love was in the dessert that we received with the Sunday meal. Love was in the first aid that we received when we had scrapes and bruises. Love was in the new dress or pants we received when all the kids at school were wearing something new. Love was in the Easter outfit that you could not wait to wear. Love was there 365 days a year and 24 hours a day whether you were receiving chastisement for wrongdoing or a hug for an achievement. Love was even in the castor oil that you had to take when anything was wrong (or sometimes before you felt something "coming on"). Love was present and we felt it. We were constantly admonished to love one another and take care of one another as siblings. The love had to continue, and it did.

In *II Timothy*, Paul encouraged Timothy to stir up the gifts that were in him. He reminded Timothy of his upbringing. *II Timothy 1:5 & 6* – "When I call to remembrance the unfeigned faith that is in thee, which dwelt first in thy grandmother Lois, and thy mother Eunice; and I am persuaded that in thee also. Wherefore I put thee in remembrance that thou stir up the gift of God, which is in thee by the putting on of my hands." I put you in remembrance of your faith. This is no new faith. This is your past, your history, and your upbringing. This is no new doctrine. It is the same doctrine your grandmother shared with your mother and the same one your mother shared with you. This is no new revelation. You are not an alien to the truth. The teachings have not left you. Search deep down within your spirit and stir up that which has been imparted. Like Timothy, we have to occasionally stir up the gift!

All of the attributes, cleanliness, allowance, responsibility, self-respect, being trustworthy, having an education, respect, family unity, pride, restrictions and love played a big part in our growing up. These attributes made us wholesome human beings with integrity, generosity and love for God and mankind. Psychologists may argue how it was applied, but they cannot argue with the results. When we learn better, we do better. I may not use the same tactics with my children, but the basic teaching still stirs within me. Mama trained us up in the ways of the Lord and it worked. None of us have departed. We are lovers of the Lord and all active in our various churches. We have never strayed long or far from Mama's teachings.

CHAPTER VIII
Communication

Communication, according to Webster, is the act of transmitting. Humans transmit messages to each other through speech: orally or by sign language; through writings: poems, books, newspaper articles, magazines, and so forth; through body language, jerks of the head, the way we sit and where (how close we get to another person), how we look at each other, all of which send messages. Satellites transmit or communicate waves to our television sets, radios and cell phones. Sunlight communicates with plant life: flowers, trees, greenery; thus they grow. Internally our brain communicates signals to our organs so that we can function. Once this information system is interrupted, communication can become slower or even halted. Dementia, namely Alzheimer's, disturbs our communication method.

Communication is a process of information exchanged. You may be grammatically incorrect, but if you are understood, then you have communicated. Babies communicate their discomfort. They do not know a language, but the message is received and interpreted of their screaming voices when they are wet or hungry. The deaf mute has a system to communicate to the speaking and hearing world even though no sound is made. Policemen have a way of communicating authority by just showing a badge or holding a piece of metal with an open barrel at the tip. Mama could look at us in church, not uttering a sound, and communicate the consequences of talking or 'acting up' during service. These consequences would be demonstrated later at home. Communication was established. We understood the message!

Communication is vital to our very existence. Verbal communication is what makes us human and distinguishes us from animals. The art of language is not known to any other species on the planet. Though other species are able to communicate, there is yet a difference in our form of verbal expression. It is a higher intelligence that causes us to listen, reason and resolve difficult situations. We can talk things out. We can listen to the counsel of the wise. We can make effective decisions. We can solve problems. We can add, subtract, divide and multiply. We can analyze situations and come up with answers to things that baffle us initially. We can decipher. We can look at past experiences and learn from them. We can take in information and store it for later usage. We can communicate through written words. We can paraphrase. We can abbreviate. We can learn new and innovative ways of doing things. We have the incredible ability to make changes when necessary.

The human brain is an awesome creation by God. We use our thinking capabilities as opposed to our instincts as some animal species will do. Sometimes the two are combined. We think and we use our instincts. Many things come naturally, but only after they have been taught or witnessed. Portions of our brains are designated for different functions. Areas of speech, memory, motor skills and language are designed to help us relate to one another and to the elements. We have opportunities to explore and learn more. We are normally complex, intelligent and reasonable beings!

How we communicate with God affects how we communicate with each other. Because of our undying faith in a God in whom we trust, we are able to accept the circumstances and search for a way to communicate with Mama. There is no placing blame. It does not matter if any one came up short in our care for her. We are now about the business of understanding what glory God can get out of the situation. We are in constant communication with Him on her behalf.

The Word of God (*Colossians 4:6*) suggests that we ought to know how to answer all men. As we decide what the best solution for a particular circumstance is, we take into account all the things that we were taught. If we are taught carnal things then our answers will be carnal responses. If we are taught spiritual things then our answers will have spiritual connotations;

which are better for us. "For to be carnally minded is death; but to be spiritually minded is life and peace." (*Romans 6:8*) What we communicate to one another comes from the spirit that lies within us. When we become 'born again' that spirit changes, but until then communication relies on what was imputed to us in our childhood. Environment, financial status, religious teachings and education direct us to either sound or impractical decisions.

As we go through life, we find ourselves constantly making decisions. Those decisions communicate to others who we are. We decide whether or not to continue our education, who we will marry, when we will start a family, what career we want to spend our time developing, whether or not we will become a Christian, and so forth and so on. Sometimes decisions may go against our will, but for our benefit. Everything belongs to God, but he does allow us free will and with that 'will' we decide some of our own fate. What has been communicated to us guides our choices whether educational, religious or political. Choose you this day which god you will serve. Will it be God or will it be Baal? We have to take into account what we have learned, what we have experienced and what we know to be true. My middle child always reminds me that we have to make a decision.

Communication starts in the home. It is a teaching process. Have you ever gone to a child's play ground and just listened to the children? You can just about determine what type of household a child comes from by the language used on the playground. You can tell in which home good grammar is taught and practiced. You can also tell who comes from a cursing family where anger is often on display or a God-fearing family where love abounds. There is a serious problem when you can spend five hours braiding a child's hair and not two hours on math, science or English. Priorities need to be set. Braided hair will not guarantee an abundant life, but a good education is a good start.

My mother was a stickler for the English language. Maybe because she knew we would have to be able to communicate properly to make it in this world. Mama did not know anything about Ebonics; she just understood that first impressions were lasting ones. She had a particular issue with the incorrect verb conjugation of 'saw' and 'seen'. It was drilled into me for as long as I can remember how to use these words. I was not allowed to mess up 'saw' and 'seen'. It made my mother cringe when they were used incorrectly. She would correct me every time. You can bet your last dollar I know how to use these two words. In fact, I am an authority on 'saw' and 'seen'. You probably saw that coming. It was seen some time ago.

Every decision we make is a culmination of our experiences, environment and education (what we have been taught). *Proverbs 22:6* states, "Train up a child in the way he should go: and when he is old, he will not depart from it." From the television shows we watch to the books we read to the movies we go to see, decisions of what should be viewed are made by what we were trained was "OK" when we were growing up. If it conflicts with what we were told was the right thing to do, then chances are we will detour from it and find another way of doing things. However, if we possess the spirit of rebellion, we find ourselves doing those things that are the opposite of what we were taught even though somewhere in the canals of our mind we know what is right. The last portion of that scripture says, "...he will not depart from it." This is to say that the training remains. The obedience may be lacking, but the training is still there.

The Game

God is the creator and owner of this world. The cattle on a thousand hills belong to God. The hills belong to God. Your money, your car, your house, your spouse, your children all belong to God. He loans these things to us. If you are willing and obedient, you can eat of the fruit of the land (Isaiah 1:19). If you are disobedient, you may be cursed. Our will is either established or broken. It is mind over matter. Another analogy: life can be compared to a tennis game. The ball is always in your court. You can serve it or you can throw it away. It is up to you; it is your will. You can pick up the ball and go with it or you can throw it in the stands. You have the option of serving the enemy with the power you possess or retreating in defeat. Match point will not be realized until you play the game.

Only the length of time that you get to play the game is out of your control. What you have to do is play well while you are on the court. You must come ready to play and play at your best. To play well you must be **physically in shape, know the rules** and you must have the **right equipment and garment**. If we look at this spiritually, God is the timekeeper. We are the players. Without the above essentials, the opponent, who is our adversary, the devil, will have the advantage. We must be spiritually in shape to play; full of the Word of God. We must also be saved, sanctified and full of the Holy Ghost. There are three essentials to playing the GAME.

(1) Be Physically In Shape

First things first: *Romans 10:9*, "That if thou shalt confess with thy mouth the Lord Jesus and shalt believe in thine heart that God hath raised him from the dead, thou shalt be saved." Regardless of your past or what you are doing at this present moment, when you confess Jesus as your Lord and Savior and believe in your heart the account from the Word of God that Jesus was crucified on the cross for your sins, buried, but rose that third day morning with all power in heaven and in earth in His hands you will be saved. We are made the righteousness of God through the blood of Jesus the Christ. Not by works, lest any man should boast, but by the saving blood of Jesus are you saved. With that blood the price of redemption was paid. If we confess it, that blood gives us life eternal with Jesus.

Paul admonished the Galatians not to allow anything or anybody to turn them from this simple truth of salvation. It is this simplicity of salvation that gets us in shape. The newly converted Jews of Galatia were being prompted to become Jewish-Christians by circumcision and keeping the law. Salvation was made difficult. Those that were issuing the edict were not keeping their own self-righteous rules. Paul encouraged the Galatians to remember what they had been taught, and to cling to the fact that Christ's blood removed the bondage of the schoolmaster. Basically, Paul was saying, walk in your salvation of which Christ has died for you. Only Jesus Christ paid the ultimate sacrifice for your eternal life with God. It was not the Pharisees or the Sadducees that gave you life. The blood of Jesus saved you. Once the Holy Ghost has come upon you, you shall receive power (*Acts 1:8*). The power of the Holy Ghost comes with that salvation. That power is to build muscles, produce stamina and render speed.

The Holy Ghost *power* allows us to lay hands on the sick and they shall recover (*Mark 16:18*). Courage and strength are needed to fight off the enemy. God did not give us the spirit of fear, but of love, power and a sound mind. You cannot cast out the spirit of sickness if you are powerless against disease because you are too 'scarred' to face the enemy. Much of our personal illnesses are due to our own conversation or lack thereof with the adversary. The power is in our tongue. According to *Proverbs 21:18*, death and life is in the power of the tongue. One of the initial program steps in Alcoholics Anonymous is confession. You must confess and confront the problem. If you never admit that you have one, you can never be healed of the disease. You will always be running from the enemy.

Stamina gives us the endurance to run the race with patience. The race is not given to the swift nor to the strong, but to the one who endures until the end. *Ecclesiastes 9:11*, "I returned, and saw under the sun, that the race is not to the swift, nor the battle to the strong, neither yet bread to the wise, nor yet riches to men of understanding, nor yet favor to men of skill; but time and chance happeneth to them all." An old cliché states that quitters never win and winners never quit. Right at the edge of the finishing line, the Holy Ghost will give that extra push to make it over into triumph. *Romans 5:3 and 4* – "And not only so, but we glory in tribulation also: knowing that tribulation worketh patience; and patience, experience; and experience, hope." This does not mean you have to endure tribulation to receive patience and therefore hope, but rather that when you are faced with tribulation, the patience that is inside of you will begin to work. Tribulation causes our patience to be activated. Every time you feel the need to give up, the Holy Ghost will empower you and start the adrenalin flowing. Through the Holy Ghost we can see the finish line.

Now *speed* quickens the Holy Spirit to give us the Word, which is sharper than any two edged sword, to fight sickness, rulers of darkness and spiritual wickedness in high places. The Word acts as our defense mechanism for safety. Right at the time He is needed, He shows up. Whether it is in a bad storm, a fiery furnace or a lion's den, God will show up right on time. In *Luke 18:7-8a*, the unsaved judge saith, "And shall not God avenge his own elect which cry day and night unto him, though he bear long with them? I tell you that he will avenge them speedily." God will come quickly and avenge the enemy when we need Him!

When you are out of the ark of safety you cannot play the game. If you are outside of the court, in the parking lot or still at home getting dressed, you cannot play the game. All players are registered and confirmed by the Registrar. A relationship has to be established between player and Registrar. He has got to know your name to give you your points. A personal contact must be made. There are no surprises. How do you get inside? *Psalm 100* tells us to enter into his gates with thanksgiving and into his courts with praise. Mama was fully equipped for the game.

(2) Know the Rules

The Bible is the rule book. *Psalm 1* – "Blessed is the man that walketh not in the counsel of the ungodly, nor stand in the way of sinners, nor sitteth in the seat of the scornful. But his delight is in the law of the Lord and in that law doth he meditate day and night." Reading is fundamental. You cannot know the rules if you do not read the rule book. During Christmas time, many a screw or bolt lay on the floor that is part of a gadget put together by dear old dad. It is actually mystical how the directions offend the man that is putting it together. He looks at the picture and commences to arrange the parts. When it is all done, extra nuts and bolts are laying there. The directions state clearly that all parts are to be used. We must read. Every book, every scripture in the Holy Bible is useful. It is for our good. Nothing is to be left out.

We have the wonderful privilege of communicating with the author of the Holy Bible. If we need to have the directions explained, we have a holy site that we can refer to. We have the privilege of prayer. We can call on God for impartation and revelation of the Word with clarity. It is essential that we study and meditate on God's Word so that we can rightly divide the Word of Truth. Whenever we are baffled by what we read, in order that we do not leave the pertinent bolts and nuts unused, God has provided the Holy Ghost to lead and guide us into all truths. When we know what God expects of us, we sin less against Him. The book of Proverbs tells us that wisdom is the principle thing, but in all of our getting - get an understanding. One of the purposes of the Holy Ghost is to give us understanding to what we read.

If the opponent knows the rules and you do not, he has the advantage. He knows when he can hit and when he needs to retreat. Victory is in knowing the rules. You must know how to combat his tactics. When he makes you feel that you have lost the game, remember it is only a part of his strategy. You have to know for yourself that the count is not out. You must look to the Time Keeper to see if the game is over. It is over only when the Time Keeper announces the end of the game. Mama's game is not over. The processing is slower, but she is not out. It may appear that she is down for the count, but it has not been called. We will wait on the Time Keeper!

Never let anyone convince you that it is over just because times are hard or the way is not clear. God never fails. If He has not declared it over – it 'ain't' over! Real faith believes God when the situation looks impossible. When it appears to be no way out and you still believe, faith is in action. Four of Job's servants delivered horrifying news of the loss of his livestock, his servants, his transportation and his family. Job's wife even suggested that he should curse his God and die. Job's friends came to his house not to comfort, but to condemn and pass judgment on him. They tried to convince Job that his troubles were due to some sin he must have committed. In all this, Job never cursed God; instead he fell to his knees and worshipped! At the end of the story Job was rewarded for his diligence and faith in God. "So the Lord blessed the latter end of Job more than his beginning..." (Job 42:12).

(3) Dress with the Right Equipment and Garment

Ephesians 6:11 - "Put on the whole armor of God, that ye may be able to stand against the wiles of the devil." Be careful to choose the right garment for the event. You cannot play tennis dressed in football gear or a fencing uniform. Being overly dressed or half dressed will cause you to lose the game. You cannot have on too much or too little. Let us not be bogged down with the sins and weights that so easily beset us, but instead we must be properly dressed with truth, the gospel of peace, faith and salvation.

When the adversary sends the first ball your way, you must have the racket in hand and ready to swing. Always be prepared to respond. Never let him catch you with your guard down. Study and keep yourself prayed up! It is a bad situation when it is your serve and you do not know the truth or you have faulty equipment. Check out your gear. Make sure there are no holes in your racket. You should not be wavering in your faith. Know the game and how to end the game that there may be peace in the stands. Believe that you will win and the victory is yours. Know that God is on your side and what ever it takes to win the game, He is Jehovah Shammah – the God that is ever present! You do not have to back up. God has promised to be with you always even unto the end of the world.

Transmission

The Kepney children had no doubt what Mama was saying; it was transmitted clearly. We knew the communication code and how to play the game. It was crystal clear. The wisdom she used was not to start communicating with us when we became teenagers, but to start praying and communicating God's will and protection for our lives at an early age. Standards were set and were adhered to consistently. Opportunities to communicate were available, but limited. We were not allowed to 'talk back'. Everything was said with respect and honor. We had to learn just how far we could go. When we learn limitations as children, it carries over into adulthood. Far too many of our young people are terminated from jobs because of a lack of respect for authority. Insubordination was not tolerated in the Kepney household. If you were a child, you acted like a child. You stayed in a child's place. When you became grown, you moved out!

To a child, chastisement is a misunderstood phenomenon. The value of it is not noticeably seen until adulthood. *Hebrews 12:5-6* states, "And ye have forgotten the exhortation which speaketh unto you as unto children; My son, despise not thou the chastening of the Lord, nor faint when thou art rebuked of him: For whom the lord loveth he chasteneth, and scourgeth every son whom he receiveth." The author is trying to make us understand that God's chastening is for our good. If ever God would remove his hand from us, we would be in grave danger. As long as we feel His hand upon us, we know that He is near and we are loved. If you endure chastening, God deals with you as a son and not as a bastard child.

After being provoked by Satan and numbering Israel, against God's wishes, and facing the dilemma of deciding his punishment, David was given three choices. He could allow seven years of famine in the land, three months before his enemies or three days pestilence in the land. David said, "I am in a great strait: let us fall now into the hand of the Lord, for his mercies are great: and let me not fall into the hand of man." *I Chronicles 21:13*. God's mercies are great and never failing. His love is so dear. It would never permanently desecrate us. It may hurt or sting a little, but it is never life threatening. Oh how He loves us!

Children do not always understand what is being communicated to them. They know that they have to accept what is being issued to them until they are grown and out of the household. It is with present understanding that we reflect on what was said and we are glad it was said. At the time we could not see the benefits, but now we are glad that our parents chastened us. It demonstrated that someone cared for our well being and was interested in how we turned out as adults. How we wish now that they could communicate those same principles to our children. Present day parenting is so different from when we were growing up in the Kepney household. It may even be considered child abuse today, but the fact remains that we are all well-adjusted adults. Mama just did what she knew to do. It never killed us!

If we fail to be good parents, it is not the fault of our mother. We have to do as Paul instructed Timothy "to stir up the gifts that is in us." He reminded Timothy that it was not a faith that started with him, but one that had been apart of his household for two generations. I know you, like Timothy, possess that same unfeigned faith. The gift of faith and knowledge, that was imputed years ago, by not only Mama, but our grandmothers as well, is like sand in an hour glass. All we have to do is flip it over and start again. The knowledge is not gone. The memories should not be forsaken. Shake it up or flip it over, but use it so that it may not go to naught.

Communication is important. Our job now is to find a way to communicate with Mama. Progress is being made in Alzheimer's research, but in case nothing significant is done in this generation, we must use simple tactics to talk with our mother. When she remembers, we must search our own Safe Places for information. We have to listen carefully and hear her heart. The words may not all fall into the right places, but the sincerity of the heart is evident. I can remember being baffled by something she said, but when I left the nursing home it came to me just what she meant.

CHAPTER IX
Healing & Peace

When we found out what was happening to Mama in medical terms, we all needed healing. Mama needed healing. Daddy needed healing and so did we -the children. We all received that healing in different ways and at different times, but we were all healed. I submit to you that the healing process begins when we let go and let God. Those things that we cannot change are to be left in the Master's hand. Because we trust Him we can accept His will for our lives and that of our loved ones. His will is that we are healed. We have to explore exactly what healing is and how we get to that place. All so familiar is the passage in Isaiah when he speaks of being healed by the stripes of Jesus. "But He was wounded for our transgressions, he was bruised for our iniquities; the chastisement of our peace was upon him and with his stripes we are healed." (*Isaiah 53:5*) What we understand that scripture to mean is the basis for our healing. The following is an explanation of that scripture.

Christ was wounded for our transgressions. The word transgression denotes a deviation from the truth. In *John 14:6*, Christ states that He is the way, the truth and the light. Any man that cometh unto the Father, must come by Him. When we deviate from what we know about Him and what He says in His Word we fall into transgression - sin. When we leave what we know to be true and the perfect will of God - we sin. We sin when we compromise the standards that God has set in His Word. Sin can be defined as 'missing the mark'.

As an archer releases his arrow from the bow, his objective is to hit the bull's eye dead in the center. There is a designated mark to hit for a score to be made. Often times he misses it. Maybe his aim is off or there exists a problem with the bow or the arrow. The target is large, but he still misses. The further he is away from the target the more difficult it appears to score. The possibility of hitting around the parameters of the mark is greater than hitting the bull's eye. Ninety-nine and a half just will not do. When we play church or just go out of duty or tradition, we hit the parameter. God requires commitment and relationship. You will never hit the eye if you do not take your time with God seriously.

Missing the mark is easy to do. *Matthew 24:24* – "For there shall arise false christs, and false prophets, and shall show great signs and wonders; insomuch that, if it were possible they shall deceive the very elect." The very elect can be standing so far to the left that even they miss the mark. Thank God for the advocate we have in Jesus Christ who was the propitiation for our sins. Christ was wounded for every time that we would miss that mark. He sits on the right hand of the Father making intercession for us when we miss the mark and confess the sin. The only way we can return from the place of transgression is to confess our sins, admit that we missed the mark, and accept His work on the cross as our redemption.

Christ was bruised for our iniquities. In other words, He was crushed, broken and oppressed for our crimes. He hung on the cross, guilty of nothing, but he took on the sins of the world to bring us back into a place of reconciliation, wholeness and oneness with God. When you need healing, you are not whole. Christ knew what it meant to be bruised. He was bruised on his way to the cross and bruised while he was there. Our spirits are often crushed, our feelings broken and our egos oppressed from sins we have committed, and those that have been committed unjustly against us, but God tells us to fear not because he has overcome the world. He has already paid the price for our iniquities and all of our shortcomings. *John 16:33* states, "These things I have spoken unto you, that in me ye might have peace. In the world ye shall have tribulation: but be of good cheer; I have overcome the world."

The chastisement of our peace was upon Him. Chastisement is correction, discipline or instruction. Peace is said to be nothing missing and nothing broken. Therefore, the correction or the reestablishing of our peace was on Christ as He hanged on the cross. When we are troubled by the calamities of life, can't sleep, can't eat or can't function we need to proceed to the foot of the cross where we can find peace. Peace is more valuable than money. You can have billions of dollars and not have peace. You can be the most popular candidate and not have peace. You may be at the top of your game, but your nights be filled with turmoil. Peace is not for sale; you cannot buy it. It comes from on High. *John 14:27* – "Peace I leave with you, my peace I give unto you: not as the world giveth, give I unto you."

Notice Christ said, "Not as the world giveth." The world's system of peace is short lived. It comes in the form of drugs, alcohol, dishonesty and loose living to name a few. All of these are temporary highs. When the high is over, you are cast down to possibly even lower depths. What goes up must come down. Only God's peace is perpetual. He promised to keep us in perfect peace if we keep our minds stayed on Him. His peace will never let you down. He also promised a peace that surpasses all understanding. Sinners will not be able to comprehend how you function when all hell has broken loose. On the outside they see your children in trouble, your power off, your spouse gone, and yet you are still smiling and yet praising God. The peace that resides on the inside shows up on the outside. Only the peace of God can cause you to stand when others would fall.

With His stripes we are healed. Every stripe Christ took on the cross was for our healing. It does not matter what the issue is – Jesus paid for it all. The stripes covered physical, financial, emotional and spiritual healing. There were upon Him stripes for diabetes, stripes for cancer, stripes for congestive heart failure, stripes for neurological disorders, stripes for addictions, stripes for mental disorders, stripes for accidents, stripes for the loss of loved ones, stripes for misunderstandings, stripes for financial disasters and stripes for dementia. These are not inclusive, the stripes covered all malfunctions of mind, body and soul. The stripes healed us and caused us to become whole. What a gruesome price He paid for us out of love.

Now the scripture states that we are healed. The 'ed' suggests the past tense. This means it is already done. The healing that we pray for is already complete in the spirit. God knew before you were conceived what was going to take place in your life. Our job is to wait on the manifestation. As we wait, we must continue to believe and praise Him like it is already done. Put your faith in God to work. Faith without works is dead. When at that point of need, you must exercise your faith and believe God. Whose report will you believe?

In Numbers 14, Moses sent 12 men to spy out the land that God had promised to them. It was an unfamiliar territory with unfamiliar inhabitants. Ten of the men came back with a negative report. "And there we saw the giants, the sons of Anak, which come of the giants: and we were in our own sight as grasshoppers, and so we were in their sights." Two men, Joshua and Caleb, came back with a positive report. "If the Lord delight in us, then he will bring us into this land, and give it us; a land floweth with milk and honey." Whose report will you believe? I choose to believe the report of the Lord.

With all that said, exactly what is healing, and how do we get there? Healing is the ability to change from an unhealthy state to a healthy state; to make sound or whole; to overcome some adversity. Matthew's accounts of Jesus' healings are many with a common denominator. To the two blind men Jesus said, "According to your **faith** be it unto you." To the woman of Canaan he said, "O woman, great is thy **faith**: be it unto thee even as thou wilt." The common denominator in each incident is 'faith'. Over and over Jesus commented on the faith of the ill; "thy faith hath made thee whole." This causes us to believe that spiritual healing requires faith either on the part of the one that is sick or the one who is standing in the gap, the mother, the father or the friend. Faith has to be put in action. All things are possible if you only believe.

How do we get to that place of healing faith? *Romans 10:17,* - "So then faith cometh by hearing, and hearing by the word of God." There is a difference between hearing and listening. As long as you listen to the Word of God, there is no application. You listen to music – no change is made in your situation. By the same token, if you just listen to the preacher – no change is made in your life. *Verse 14* in that same chapter reads: "How then shall they call on him in whom they have not believed? And how shall they believe in him of whom they have not heard? And how shall they hear without a preacher?" It profits you nothing if you listen to the preacher Sunday after Sunday and never use the powerful message that you hear. The Word will work for you, but only if you apply it. You must HEAR the Word!

Hearing requires a sincere desire to receive the Word. If what you listen to does not change any area of your life upon application, then you are listening to respond as opposed to listening to learn. It is when we realize that we do not know it all and we place ourselves in a position to be taught that we begin to hear. It is at this time that what enters the ear canal is actually received through the necessary brain stem and we begin to make changes. Application is essential to growth. If you never apply what you learn, it will never be useful to you. When you do the same thing the same old way you get the same results.

Once you begin to hear, you hear not only with your ears, but also with your heart and soul. It becomes a part of you. You act on what you hear. The Word becomes applicable to your lifestyle. For every situation, there is a scripture; there are instructions and guidance. There is nothing new under the sun. The man at the pool of Bethesda listened to what people were saying about the healing of the water, but never acted on what he heard, so he laid there some 38 years. Jesus asked him, "Wilt thou be made whole?" We think quite naturally that if someone has been sick for that long that he would want to be healed. Jesus knew that with healing comes responsibility. Do you really want to be healed, or do you just want to continue to depend on the kindness and mercy of others? After 38 years, I would have found a way to roll into the pool. We can become comfortable and complacent in our infirmity. Christ said that He came that we might have life and it more abundantly. Abundance does not include sickness. It includes healing of my body, my emotions, my issues, my finances, my family, and my life.

The woman with the issue of blood heard about Jesus. She suffered for 12 years. Luke said she went to several doctors and spent all she had. She sought after first, second, third and probably more opinions regarding her conditions. She could not find a solution. When she had had enough, and only when she had had enough, she acted on what she heard. She had been listening to the talk about Jesus and His healing the infirmed. It is when she 'heard' that the healing was available to her that she sought Jesus. All she had to do was to seek the Healer. She did just that, letting nothing hinder her quest. Scripture says that she said within herself, "If I but could touch the hem of his garment I would be made whole." The woman pressed her way through the crowd and made contact with the healer. His response was, "Daughter, be of good comfort: thy faith hath made thee whole; go in peace."

"For a certain woman, whose young daughter had an unclean spirit, heard of him, and came and fell at his feet..." (*Mark 7:25*). The scripture states that, "She heard of him." This woman had a child that was sick. The nurturing spirit within a woman will cause her to search to the ends of the earth for help for her children. She knew there was healing somewhere for her child and she heard about a healer named Jesus. He was in an undisclosed house that no man knew, but she found Him. When we are serious about our pursuit for an answer we will do whatever is necessary to find it. She put her faith in action. Even when it appeared she was receiving rejection from Jesus, she continued to pursue healing for her child. Her victory came because she would not give up. Jesus declared in verse *29*, "...For this saying go thy way, the devil is gone out of thy daughter." Her child was healed.

Let us explore another example of putting faith into action. In the 7th chapter of *II Kings,* there is a story of four leprous men sitting outside of a city gate. They had been ostracized because of their disease. In the third verse they said, "Why sit we here until we die?" A decision had to be made. We can either sit here and die or go into the city. If there is a famine in the city and we die, we die, but at least we made an effort to live. God expects us to do something with our belief. In Hebrews, the Scripture says they entered not into the rest of God because of their unbelief. God can put our belief to the test. He needs to know that we believe what we confess and that we accept the responsibility of our confessions. If you believe God to be a healer, and you confess it, you must also live it.

If we believe in healing, we must walk in our healing and not make foolish decisions. If we have trouble with high blood pressure, it is foolish to eat pork and salt on a daily basis. If the medical report states we have diabetes, it is foolish to eat ice cream every day. This brings us back to the word responsibility. We must act responsibly with God's blessings. Will you be made whole?

As I alluded to earlier, healing takes on different forms. It may be total recovery, comfort from pain, or even death. While Mama's communication skills are hindered, her body is sustained and her soul is healed. Her family has to make the adjustment and heal from our emotional wounds. There is no one to blame. We must heal. We must trust God's predestinated plan for our lives. We must heal. The only way to go forward is to heal of your present and your past circumstances. We have to make a decision to be healed.

CHAPTER X
The Mind:
A Terrible Thing to Lose

The Negro College Fund has a popular saying, "The mind is a terrible thing to waste." I agree, but it is also a terrible thing to lose. As a man thinks in his heart, so is he. Out of the heart come the issues of life. These Bible scriptures do not refer to the organ that pumps blood, but rather the mind, which as a former pastor of mine used to say, is the seed of your intellect. The mind is what thinks, calculates and recalls. Losing control of its function leaves us at the mercy of others. It becomes death to us and an additive to the caretaker.

It is one thing to experience the lengthy illness of a loved one and another to experience a sudden tragic death. A lengthy illness gives you time to prepare. It gives you time to accept what God has allowed. You can develop a strategy against the enemy. A plan is put into place and whatever it takes, you have to pull yourself together and do what is necessary. Sure, you may shed tears. You may ask why, but you still have to find out what has to be done and do it. You move on because life goes on. You tend to the needs of the loved one and prepare yourself for the inevitable.

In an unexpected fatal occurrence, there is no time to say goodbye. When death is sudden, everything that should have been said, if not said when the opportunity presented itself, has to be left unsaid. Feelings of guilt fester. The wish that we had done so many things differently manifests. If only there was some more time. We take advantage of time, not realizing that we do not own time. We do not know how long we will have with those who are so dear to us. Tomorrow is not promised to us. Therefore, we should cherish every waking moment.

Do not let the sun go down on your wrath. Resolve issues before you close your eyes. Paul wrote to the Church at *Ephesus* in chapter *4*, verse *26*: "Be ye angry, and sin not: let not the sun go down upon your wrath." It is human nature to get angry. There is not one person alive who could admit to never becoming angry. There are those of us who have better control over our wrath and demonstrate more temperance than others. There are those of us who have no control. Paul says to be angry and sin not. He did not say, 'but sin not' rather he said 'and sin not'. This lets us know that we are going to become angry, but we can and should exercise control.

Always express warm feelings toward friends and family. Expressions of love are never too numerous. Even the utterance of those so infrequently used words, "I Love You", can make a difference in the life of a child, a spouse, a mother, a father, sister or brother. Just knowing that you care and want to understand what is going on in the life of another gives a sense of security. Never let a loved one assume how you feel about them. Take the initiative and say it first. Watch the instant Kodak moment you will receive.

Alzheimer's does not give you that option. It attacks, and the victim is oftentimes unaware of what is happening. It creeps into the mind so subtly that only those who have witnessed it before can tell what is going on. It is cruel and devastating. It leaves the caretaker with thoughts of, "If I had only known, I would have..." The truth of the matter is that you do not know until the symptoms become irreversible. All you can do is cope with the situation. Coping takes some education. You have to be educated about the disease, what to expect and how to handle the prognosis. Alzheimer's can cause us to step into a world so different from our own that we find ourselves bewildered and not knowing which way to turn. We ask, "How did this happen?" "Why did this happen?"

CHAPTER XI
My Mother/My Friend

My mother is my friend. It was a long journey to that friendship. I was the typical teenager that felt misunderstood, believing that Mama and Daddy did not know what they were talking about. They just did not understand, because they were too old. So I passed through the stages of rebellion. I wanted to have my way, and no one was going to stop me. Going away to college meant freedom, so I thought (it would get me out of the house). What it brought outside of the education was trouble after trouble after trouble. Guess who was there through it all to bail me out? That is right, it was Mama.

It was not until I married and had my family that my mother and I really developed any intimacy. It was then that I begin to understand the parent-to-child relationship. In the eyes of a child, the adult figure is often the enemy. All of the good that is done goes unnoticed. It is taken for granted. The attitude is "You are supposed to do things for me". The child notices the negative and rarely concentrates on the positive. As adults we reflect on the nurturing, the caring and love that we received. The chastisement was good for us. We could not see it then, but maturing brings you to a complete awareness of just how good life was.

True friendship is difficult to find. Friends share without ceasing. They call with nothing specific to talk about, but just to say 'hello' or to ask 'how are you doing'. Friends share not only the big things, and the minute things that mean so much, but even things that do not have any value at all. Friends share good news and bad. They share births, graduations and weddings. Friends share accidents, pain and funerals. They love unconditionally. They talk and listen when necessary. They comfort and discipline each other. They agree and they disagree. Through it all they remain friends. Mama and I are friends.

How I wish I could reach that part of Mama's brain to remind her who I am and what we mean to each other! As I watch her search for words or bring up totally unrelated events, I search for the right word or phrase myself that would trigger some fun memory of our friendship. The root word of relationship, of course, is the word 'relate'. We had reached that point of sincere relationship. I knew that I could say almost anything to her, and the judgment would be different. We were able to relate to each other. She shared intimate things that I never knew about her; things that were so very personal. She had become comfortable with me, and I with her. The mother/daughter wall had been torn down and a wall of mother/daughter/friend had replaced it. It was like a chain link fence that you could add to forever.

We had many conversations. We talked about life, husbands, church issues, work and children. We never talked about each other (after all it was a long distance call and we just did not have time for that). As the oldest, I was privileged to help evaluate the lives of my younger siblings. In our discussions, of course, I understood where Mama was coming from where they were concerned, because I was the oldest. I really just enjoyed talking about my brother and sisters and finding out what was going on in their lives!

It is interesting how the age gap closes as you get older. I have friends who are 10 and 15 years younger than I am. I would not have even considered making them a part of my world when I was in the twelfth grade and they were not even in middle school! As we experience life, our environments become mutual. We may not take the same route, but the destination is the same. We have the same wilderness experiences which brings us closer together. People relate better to other people when they have shared things in common. After some bumps and turns, I could understand Mama's reasonings in some areas; whereas before it did not make sense. I guess you can say time and experience brought us closer.

Mama and I were proud of each other. When I would come home, Mama would have a calendar loaded with engagements. She would take me along, so that she could introduce me to her colleagues. She would introduce me as her 'Oldest' who had graduated from college and lived in Alabama. She was so proud. I got to know how she really felt when she had the opportunity of introducing me before a church group in Houston. She said things that warmed my heart.

I was equally proud of her. Mama was my role model as a parent, a wife, and a speaker. When I became a mother, she came in quite handy. Her phone might ring in the middle of the night, from a daughter who needed to know what to do with this 'crying baby'. Mama was always ready with an answer. As a wife, she taught me to honor the head of the house and respect his position. As a speaker, she taught the unadulterated truth of God. She studied so that she would not be ashamed because she could rightly divide the Word of God.

When I see a smile that just comes out of nowhere, I want to believe it is a fun memory of days gone by and of a relationship that shall never end. She will forever be my friend. Though separated by miles and intellect, we are not separated in spirit. I trust that God will grant me the desire of my heart: that my mother will be at peace and happy with the thoughts she has that so often go verbally unexpressed. I pray that she will someday remember who she is in Him and know that the peace she experiences is of God. I want her to feel His presence; to know that He is forever with her. Even if she cannot tell us, I pray that somewhere in the canals of her mind that she knows that she is kept by God!

CHAPTER XII
What Do We Do With Mama?

Our initial response to what was happening to the pillar of strength of the family was to deny. Denial is a long road to nowhere. After you detour, take a turn; make a left and then a right, you still have the problem. It hinders you from doing the inevitable. Denial is a waste of precious time. It places you in a no win situation. Denial was our demon. It haunted us until we made a decision. *James 4:7* – "Submit yourselves therefore to God. Resist the devil, and he will flee from you." This does not mean to run, but to face your enemy and he will run from you. In school, as long as you ran from a bully, he would continue to taunt you and threaten you daily. He may have run you home from school until the day came that you had enough! You turned around and faced him. If you are running from the devil, you will never win. It is only when you stop and face the enemy, and confront the problem that victory will occur. Face him with the Word of God, and he has to flee. Mama has a form of dementia. We can face it or keep running. What do we do?

At Christmas time, it was the norm for Mama to do most or all of the cooking. She baked the turkey and the ham, fixed the macaroni and cheese, the dressing, the greens and the corn bread. She was famous for her German Chocolate Cake. The cake alone would take her half of the day to complete. She made it from scratch. I would put that cake up against anybody's. It was sure to win the best cake contest. We loved to eat it while it was still hot, fresh out of the oven. After cutting the cake, it was gone within a few hours of its manifestation. We would hide it from visitors! We were trying to save it just for the immediate family. We would actually wait until they left the premises before slicing the cake. It was just that good!

The Christmas when the dementia demon showed him self, I did not want to admit that something was wrong. I saw clear signs, but continued to deny. The most obvious was the preparing of the Christmas dinner and the German Chocolate Cake. Mama laid out all of the necessary ingredients and the pans needed for the baking of the cake. She had melted the chocolate for the icing and placed it on the counter. She took a pot off of the stove and placed it inside of the pot with the melted chocolate. The bottom of the pot was covered with chocolate. She then took the coconut that would be used for the icing and started to make the corn bread for the dressing out of it. When I noticed what she was doing, I immediately offered to make the corn bread. Though still in denial, the rest of the siblings pitched in to complete the Christmas feast. Under our watchful eye, we allowed her to cook some of the food, but we were careful to say grace before eating. Needless to say the German Chocolate Cake never materialized. I regrettably suffered it to be so!

God is yet good. Dementia in its initial stages will allow your mind to come and go. During that same Christmas gathering, Mama called me to her bedroom and gave me an envelope that contained her wishes upon her demise. She had written it long ago and knew that this was the time to give it to the oldest. (Look at God; He is still in charge!) I took the envelope with tears in my eyes, but I knew it had to be done. I did not share this with my siblings because they were in a worse state of denial than I was. I just tucked it in my suitcase to take back home and put in a secure place until the time was right.

Mama also informed me that she wanted me to return to Shreveport for another visit during the week when the banks and business offices were open so that we could get important papers signed. She wanted my name on legal matters to prevent confusion in the future. This is crucial. If your elderly loved ones are yet in their right minds, take advantage of the situation and get important legal matters established: power of attorney, guardianship, and living wills. I never returned to do that, maybe because I was in denial or just did not want to do it. When our father passed, I remembered that conversation with Mama and regretted not following through.

Talks with my father, let us know that other things had been going on that he did not understand. Mama went into the kitchen at 2:00 o'clock one morning and began cooking dinner. Daddy had a hard time convincing her to come back to bed. He noticed that her memory was gradually getting away from her. She drove to her hair salon, one that she had used for more than 20 years, and when done called him to pick her up. The car was in the parking lot of the salon. Daddy said she would go to the grocery store, stay away for hours and would come back home with no groceries. Mama had started wandering. Her mind would not settle in one place for a long period of time. All these things were signs that something was wrong.

Dementia gradually gets worse. More memory is lost, and conversations become very strange. Names, directions, courtesies, personal hygiene and things that we take for granted disappear. Simple things like putting clothes and shoes on or combing the hair become an ordeal for the sufferer. It may go from, "Where are my shoes?" to "Why can't I remember how to put my shoes on?" There seems to be a common need to "go home". Mama always wanted to go home. Home is always remembered. Now, it may be the most recent home or the home from childhood, but it represents a *'Safe Place'*.

Finally, when my father accepted that Mama's care was beyond what he could do, he called us in for a family council. We had to make a decision. We had to come out of denial. We had to face the facts. I must put a pin right here. Regardless of what is happening to our dear mother, God has the final answer. There is a great difference between 'fact' and 'truth'. Fact says that you are ill, but the Truth says by His stripes you are healed. Fact says that the money is out and the bills are due, Truth says he will supply all of our needs according to His riches in glory. Fact says that the children are out of control and the husband is unsaved, the Truth says train up a child in the way he should go and when he is old he will not depart and that a woman can sanctify her husband and cause her household to be Holy. You weigh the scale; will it be FACT or TRUTH that you choose to believe?

Mama's physician led us into acceptance with much resistance. Surely there is a pill for this. Is this temporary? Daddy overwhelmed him with questions that we all needed answered: will it get any better, is there any medication she can take, how did this happen? Can we take her home? Is this terminal? Who will she remember? Will she ever remember me again? Again, we had to escape denial. What do we do?

Elderly people suffering from dementia need full time care. Daddy maintained a part- time job as a crossing guard and as janitor of his church. He did not want to give them up. There were outstanding bills existing in the household, that he felt he had to work to pay. He would not be able to manage the job, the house, his church work and Mama. We did not want the burden on him because he had health issues himself. All of us had jobs and children in school. We decided, with much regret, to place Mama in a nursing facility that accepts dementia patients. That was difficult. Dementia patients are hard to place because of the big risk factor. The problem of wandering off to another location away from the facility was an issue. Many nursing homes do not have a lock down facility where dementia patients can be cared for, and some simply do not want to be bothered. However, we did eventually, by the Grace of God, find a very nice facility. It was not too far from home and Daddy could visit regularly.

We were all there for the early stages of the move. It broke our hearts. We tried to give her room a familiarity of home; with pictures, whatnots and anything that would remind her of us. Daddy bought her a television with a remote. We bought new comfortable clothing. We put her name in and on personal items; to no avail. On a return visit most of the items we brought from home were missing. It was not the fault of the nursing home, Mama had carried things to different parts of the home and the caretakers could not figure out what belonged to whom. The remote was as in any typical remote at the house– lost. Mama would put on any shoe that did not have a pair of feet in them. Clothes she stuffed in her drawers may or may not belong to her. Pictures were moved or missing. This took some getting used to.

When everything was moved in, we gathered to talk with her. We prayed with her. We kissed and hugged her. She seemed to enjoy the attention. We loved on her, but we had to leave her. She pleaded with us not to leave. She, like us, could not understand why we had to leave her in this unfamiliar place. She just wanted to go home. Where is home? We had to maneuver our departure by leaving the room one by one. Crying as we left, we had to go. We did not want to leave her there. We wanted her back in the kitchen humming a spiritual song as she cooked for us, her family. We wanted to see her all dressed up for church. We longed to see her sitting on the side of the bed as she read the Word of God so that she could impart spiritual revelations to some class or congregation. We would welcome the fussing if we could take her back home. I can still hear her pleas. "Don't go" rings in my ears even now. What do you do?

CHAPTER XIII
The Conclusion of the Matter

SO, WHAT DO WE DO WHEN BAD THINGS HAPPEN TO GOD'S CHOSEN? Where is the Safe Place? The answer is quite simple, but it takes years to realize. Whom God calls, He qualifies. All the wonderful insights that God yielded to Mama did not go unnoticed. They are not futile. What God instilled in her she used, and she benefited from it, others benefited from it as well and so did we. Physically, she is still with us, and we thank God for that. Mentally, she is in a *Safe Place* that is inaccessible to us. Our prayer has been to keep her in peace and good health. God has answered our prayer. Except for minor physical problems that are being controlled by medication and good care, she is doing well. Sometimes she calls our names correctly and we think positively because we want to believe that she recognizes us. She still smiles. She continues to make funny comments. The personality is still there, untouched by the enemy who tried to take her mind. Like Isaiah asked in the 57th chapter, "How do we know that God did not allow this, to keep her from a greater evil that was yet to come her way?"

We cannot be bitter about what has happened to Mama. She is really at peace with nothing missing and nothing broken. Peace is more important to the human spirit than any emotional element that you can acquire. Peace is more valuable than money. Mama has peace. There are sane people who do not know what they are doing or what they are supposed to do or what their purpose is. They do not know whether to turn left or right. Mama has peace. Some wealthy people cannot sleep at night for worrying about how to make more money. Mama has peace. There are educated people who cannot decide whether to continue in school or get a job. Mama is at peace. Some have to decide which utility to pay because the last paycheck was not sufficient. Should we pay the power bill or the phone bill? Mama has peace. No more worries, no concerns – just peace that surpasses all understanding.

"Thou wilt keep him in perfect peace, whose mind is stayed on thee: because he trusteth in thee." *(Isaiah 26:3)* Perfect peace can only be obtained when you trust in God. Mama has always trusted in God. She does not know not to trust Him. Before things changed, she trusted him. Who is to say that trust does not remain? God is keeping her in a perfect peace that is beyond our comprehension. She does not exhibit any anxiety, pain or a disturbed spirit. The only thing that is visible is a quiet spirit and an uplifted countenance. Look at God! He is not only good to her, but He is good to us. He allows us to experience peace of mind, just knowing that Mama is at peace.

Therefore, the answer to the question, "What do we do", is what Mama continually taught us – "Trust in God." The only reason *Isaiah 57:1* can be comforting to us, is because we trust God. When you cannot trace Him, you must still trust Him. Many times when we felt forsaken, with Mama's condition and Daddy gone, we were at a place in God where we asked the question 'WHY'? We know that before the foundation of the world, God knew this day would come. He has a plan for our lives. *Jeremiah 29:11* tells us that he knows our end before our actual beginning. "I know the thoughts I have toward you. They are thoughts of peace and not evil to get you to an expected end." God knows who we are, how we are and how much we can bear. We can trust Him. We have to persevere. My Grandmother Laura used to say, "I believe I'll run on and see what the end 'gon' be!"

Salvation

Salvation is so important to God that He allows whatever means necessary to get you to that expected end. What is the expected end? God desires a relationship with you. He prefers that we are reconciled from this world of sin to be close to Him. From the beginning of time God devised means of restoring what was lost in the Garden of Eden – the relationship with Him. When man sinned, he separated himself from God. Sin separates us from God. God is so merciful that He allows us to return to him unconditionally. He desires that no one would perish. With love and kindness, He has drawn us in spite of ourselves. While we were yet sinners and ungodly, Christ died for us. As prodigal sons, we returned. God was waiting with a coat, a ring and a party held in our honor. What a mighty God we serve!

The answer to the question "**WHAT DO WE DO WHEN BAD THINGS HAPPEN TO GOD'S CHOSEN**" lies in our acceptance of the salvation that is available to all. It lies in trusting in a God whom we have never seen, but we can have a personal relationship with as Father and Child. It lies in believing the Word of God and applying it to our everyday lives. The answer is within us. It is a choice that we have to accept or deny. Actually, it is a choice to trust or give up! The loved one affected cannot afford for us to give up. It is just unacceptable. It is not a solution. With so many resources of help available, there is no need to throw in the towel. We must continue to avail ourselves to Him who is El Shaddai; the all sufficient one, the God who is more than enough; that we may be positioned to learn and receive understanding of the unfamiliar.

We will hold on to the memories as precious stones. No one can take away those memories. For Mama, they might not fall in chronological order, but they are there. So they are very safe. Now when she brings up a thought or a person's name that has been long gone, we will just smile and say, "Oh yea, I think I can remember." Some day we will. We can share those moments now with our spouses, our children, our siblings, and our friends, or with who ever will listen. Good memories make for marvelous stories of entertainment for both the young and old. The older you get, the more you have. The more you have, the more you can share.

Mama is a chosen vessel of God. I will forever remember her as a strong woman who fought for her family until the war was over. She was armed and dangerous. She was well dressed for battle. Mama wore the whole armor of God. Her loins were girt about with truth. She wore the breastplate of righteousness. Her feet were shod with the preparation of the gospel of peace. She had a shield of faith. She humbly wore the helmet of salvation while she carried the sword of the Spirit, which is the Word of God. Most important of all is that she passed on that armor that it may shield her offspring. She knew that the battle was not going to end with her, so she prepared the soldiers that were to become behind her. Mama dressed us with a spiritual armor that only God can provide.

It was sometimes a physical war that she fought. She engaged in mental wars and often spiritual wars as well. Whatever battle took place, in the end Mama WON! Hallelujah, she won! We have to keep in mind, that the end of a Christian's story is 'we win'. If we ever realize just who we are in Christ, our battles will not seem so insurmountable. Greater is he that is in us, than he that is in the world. We win. There is nothing too hard for God. There is nothing that God and I cannot handle together. I am victorious through Christ Jesus. He is Jehovah Nissi. He is the banner of righteousness on which I stand. He goes before me and shields me from danger. With Him all things are possible. God has never lost a battle.

You ask, "How can a person who is now in a nursing home have won the battle?" I am glad you asked. Her last thoughts of Jesus were that He lives and He saves. Like the Hebrew boys she will die knowing that God is able! We cannot change what is already there. We cannot take away the memories or the knowledge she received. It is there in her '***Safe Place'.*** What we learn and accept can be embedded in our spirits so much so that it just becomes natural. It is natural for Mama to believe God. It is as natural as breathing. No one has to tell her to breathe, she just breathes. Without realizing what was happening in her mind, Mama naturally believed God. That never changed. She did not curse God or hold Him in account. She trusted Him then and in some strange way, she trusts Him now.

My father-in-law was victim to Alzheimer's as well. His actions were a little more forceful, but they were the result of the same degenerative disease. Bro. James White was very active in his church. He was a deacon and the Sunday school superintendent. He loved the church and the work he was assigned. He was one of the devotion leaders that could really 'raise' a hymn. After he had suffered about a year, I helped him to go to a prayer meeting held at the church. We decided to give him an opportunity to sing a hymn. The same man that we could not reach with a simple conversation led the hymn without missing one note or lyric. Somewhere in his 'Safe Place' he tucked the hymns he loved so well. When the chance came, he reached into his Safe Place, found a hymn and sung his song. Look at God!

None of the Bible lessons Mama taught, the Sunday School Reviews she gave, and the Women's Day programs where she spoke were in vain. Nothing was lost. Nothing was without value. Somebody learned from her. Someone's destiny was changed from a life of destruction to a full life in Christ. Some mother was encouraged to not give up. Some father realized the end was not yet and that there was a God who cared. Some children did not succumb to the pressure of their peers. Some elderly person found the will to live. Somebody was saved and is now living in the fullness of his righteousness and not beneath his privilege.

All this was accomplished because of Mama's efforts. Her life is valuable. She has done a good work for God. The enemy has not stopped trying to pervert her family, but what she has demonstrated as a Christian woman lives on in us. He has no authority over the Kepney clan! We have been endowed with knowledge and knowledge is power!

Mama has scored. She has made first chair. Match point was made. She has been wife, mother and friend. She has taught well. Now, she can retrieve and enjoy sweet memories from her '**Safe Place**'!

APPENDIX

TIPS FOR COMMUNICATING WITH A PERSON WITH DEMENTIA

1) Show a positive attitude and mood. Be pleasant, respectful, and affectionate.

2) Get the person's attention. Turn off the TV or radio to avoid distractions.

3) Use simple words and short sentences to state your message clearly.

4) Ask simple, answerable questions. Yes or no questions work best.

5) Listen to body language as well as words. Your loved one could be struggling for words.

6) Break activities down into steps.

7) If your loved one gets upset try to change the subject or activity quickly.

8) Use affection and reassurance. Your loved one could be confused or unsure of them selves.

9) Ask about the distant past, "The good old days".

10) Use humor when possible.

Medicine Partners
Post Office Box 2628
Pflugerville, TX 78691
August 2004 Issue Page 2

Jude 24-26

Now unto Him
That is able to keep you from
falling, and to Present you faultless
before the presence of His Glory
with exceeding joy,
To the only wise God our Savior,
Be glory and majesty, dominion
and power,
Both now and ever.
Amen!

ABOUT THE BOOK

Are you experiencing the lost of someone you love
that has fallen prey to dementia; namely Alzheimer's?
Are you unsure of what the next step is? Do you yearn
for answers? Be aware, you are not alone.

This book is designed to share with its readers the
emotions, the struggles and some solutions to what
can devastate a family when a member has been
issued this fate. You will come to realize that there is
a 'Safe Place' for each victim. You can find comfort in
knowing that there is one who cares about you and
your loved one. It is all in getting an understanding of
who God is and what the disease is all about.

Though I do not claim to know all of the answers,
you will find similar situations that compare to your
own and how my father, siblings and I handled the
challenges. "A Safe Place for Mama" was written with
sudden burst of laughter and occasional warm tears
of painful memories while being assured that God is in
charge of it all. You will learn to trust Him. It can bring

you closer to the loved one as you begin to unravel mysteries and accept realities. It will bring you closer to God as your trust and your faith in Him increases.

It is my strong desire that as you read this book, you will be inspired and strengthened to face the unfamiliar; remembering that there is nothing too hard for God!

May you find a peace that will surpass all understanding!